# Flexible Sigmoidoscopy

# Flexible Sigmoidoscopy

**Douglas K. Rex, MD, FACP, FACG**
Professor of Medicine
Indiana University School of Medicine
Director of Endoscopy
Indiana University Hospital
Indianapolis, Indiana

**Blair S. Lewis, MD**
Associate Clinical Professor of Medicine
Mount Sinai School of Medicine
New York, New York

Blackwell
Science

*Blackwell Science*

Editorial Offices:
238 Main Street, Cambridge,
Massachusetts 02142, USA
Osney Mead, Oxford OX2 0EL,
England
25 John Street, London WC1N
2BL, England
23 Ainslie Place, Edinburgh EH3
6AJ, Scotland
54 University Street, Carlton,
Victoria 3053, Australia
Arnette Blackwell SA, 1 rue de
Lille, 75007 Paris, France
Blackwell Wissenschafts-Verlag
GmbH
Kurfürstendamm 57, 10707
Berlin, Germany
Feldgasse 13, A-1238 Vienna,
Austria

Distributors:
*North America*
Blackwell Science, Inc.
238 Main Street
Cambridge, Massachusetts 02142
(Telephone orders: 800–215–1000 or
617–876–7000)

*Australia*
Blackwell Science Pty Ltd
54 University Street
Carlton, Victoria 3053
(Telephone orders: 03–347–5552)

*Outside North America and
Australia*
Blackwell Science, Ltd.
c/o Marston Book Services, Ltd.
P.O. Box 87
Oxford OX2 0DT
England
(Telephone orders: 44–1865–791155)

Acquisitions: Christopher Davis
Development: Debra Lance
Production: Karen Feeney
Manufacturing: Kathleen Grimes

Printed and bound by Maple-Vail,
Binghamton, NY

© **1996 by Blackwell Science, Inc.**

Printed in the United States of
America

96  97  98  99  5  4  3  2  1

*Library of Congress Cataloging in Publication Data*

Rex, Douglas K.
    Flexible sigmoidoscopy / Douglas K. Rex, Blair S. Lewis.
        p.   cm.
    Includes bibliographical references and index.
    ISBN 0-86542-369-5 (pbk.)
    1. Sigmoidoscopy.  I. Lewis, Blair S.  II. Title.
    [DNLM:  1. Sigmoidoscopy—methods.
    2. Sigmoidoscopy—instrumentation.  WI 620 R455f 1996]
RC804.S47R49   1996
617.5'547—dc20
DNLM/DLC
for library of Congress                                95-22330
                                                          CIP

# Contents

▼ ▼ ▼ ▼ ▼ ▼ ▼ ▼

▼
▼

# Preface

▼　▼　▼　▼　▼　▼　▼　▼

T HE INTENDED AUDIENCE for *Flexible Sigmoidoscopy* is non-colonoscopists who want to acquire skills or improve their skills in flexible sigmoidoscopy. Although this audience will be comprised mainly of primary care physicians, physicians' assistants and nurses have also developed proficiency in flexible sigmoidoscopy.

This book is not an exhaustive discussion of the literature on either flexible sigmoidoscopy or colorectal pathology. Primary care physicians are busy people who must keep up with a remarkably diverse and expanding body of medical knowledge. Therefore we have tried to make this book short enough that a primary care physician could actually find the time to read it. *Flexible Sigmoidoscopy* covers the essentials of flexible sigmoidoscopy, from setting up the room to performing the examination in a safe and competent fashion. In order to make the book both useful and practical, we have tried to address all of the clinically pertinent issues that arise in regard to routine flexible sigmoidoscopy, while summarizing the relevant literature in controversial areas, rather than presenting all sides of an issue in exhausting detail.

Although a digital rectal examination must be performed on every patient undergoing flexible sigmoidoscopy, it is not necessary for the examiner to be an expert in anorectal disease. The indication for flexible sigmoidoscopy is often an anorectal symptom, however, and examiners may choose to use Chapter 5, which discusses anorectal evaluation and disease, to enhance their ability to understand, identify, and treat anorectal disease.

For readers who want more extensive information, each chapter is followed by a list of annotated selected references.

Our fundamental purpose for writing this book is that endoscopic screening of the colon for adenomas and cancer offers the most powerful tool currently available to prevent deaths from colorectal cancer. Although many people are still dying from colorectal cancer, recent studies show that there is now great hope that this can be changed. Sigmoidoscopy is not an appealing procedure to the public, however, and may not lend itself to mass screening. In all likelihood the success of sigmoidoscopic screening will depend on the extent to which it is performed by primary care givers. More than with any other physician, patients develop a long-standing relationship of trust and friendship with their primary care givers. This trust forms the basis by which a thorough primary care physician can perform sigmoidoscopic screening in patients. We believe this book will help the interested primary care giver develop skill in sigmoidoscopy, and we know that screening sigmoidoscopy will prevent deaths from colorectal cancer. Good luck!

Douglas K. Rex
Blair S. Lewis

**Notice:** The indications and dosages of all drugs in this book have been recommended in the medical literature and conform to the practices of the general medical community. The medications described do not necessarily have specific approval by the Food and Drug Administration for use in the diseases and dosages for which they are recommended. The package insert for each drug should be consulted for use and dosage as approved by the FDA. Because standards of usage change, it is advisable to keep abreast of revised recommendations, particularly those concerning new drugs.

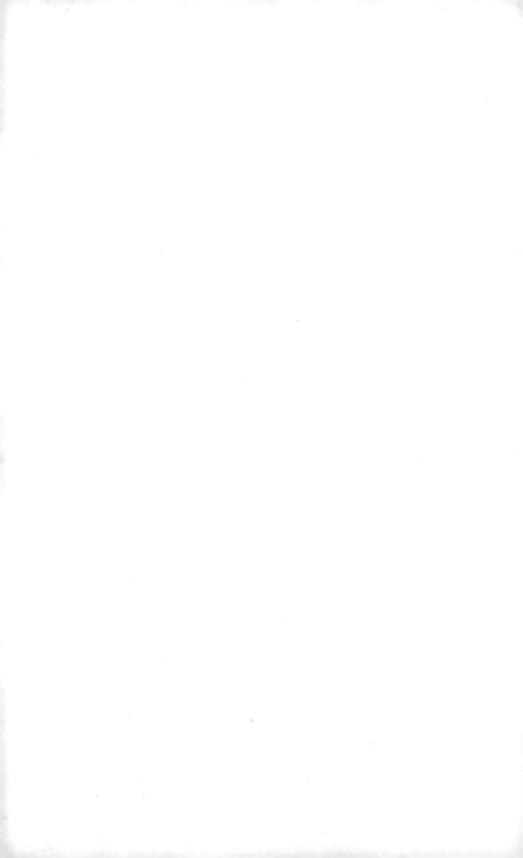

# Instruments and Office Needs

▼    ▼    ▼    ▼    ▼    ▼    ▼    ▼

## ■ FUNDAMENTALS OF INSTRUMENT DESIGN

The first decision in purchasing a sigmoidoscope often is whether to buy a fiberoptic flexible sigmoidoscopy system or a video system. For the purpose of performing a complete examination and obtaining all necessary specimens, both systems are perfectly adequate. The only advantage of fiberoptic systems is that they are substantially less expensive. A very acceptable fiberoptic system can be purchased for under $7,000. The main advantage of video systems for the primary care physician may be that the patient is able to watch the examination. Patients often are very impressed by the examination and may be more likely to follow-up on findings, and the video system may become something of a self-marketing tool as patients discuss their experience with friends and family. The video system also facilitates assistant participation in the procedure, produces less fatigue and neck strain in the examiner if multiple examinations are performed, and allows for a range of options for recording endoscopic images. Nevertheless, video systems are a substantially greater financial investment than fiberoptic systems, with the purchase price for sigmoidoscope, light source, and processor typically in the $35,000 range (Tables 1.1, 1.2, and 1.3). Welch-Allyn offers a "proximal video camera" for approximately $4,000 that, when coupled with the inexpensive FX-100 flexible sigmoidoscope, allows video tape recording and still photography. Thus, this is the least expensive video system available, but not the highest quality. Several companies offer video convertors that will capture the image of a fiberoptic scope and convert it to a video image. However, these

**1**
▼

**Table 1.1** *Light Sources for Fiberoptic and Video Sigmoidoscopes*

| Manufacturer/Model | Bulb | Watts | Price (U.S.) (6/1/94) |
|---|---|---|---|
| Fujinon | | | |
| PS2HP | Halogen | 150 | $995 |
| FLX2000 | Xenon | 300 | $8700 |
| Olympus | | | |
| CLK-4 | Halogen | 150 | $820 |
| CLE-10 | Halogen | 150 | $3500 |
| XLS | Xenon | 175 | $4680 |
| CLE-F10 | Halogen | 150 | $6330 |
| CLV-U20 | Xenon | 300 | $9060 |
| CLV-F10 | Xenon | 300 | $21,100 |
| Pentax | | | |
| LH-150P | Halogen | 150 | $820 |
| LH-150FP | Halogen | 150 | $2100 |
| LX-3000 | Xenon | 300 | $8900 |
| Welch-Allyn | | | |
| LX-150 | Halogen | 150 | $778* |

In general, xenon light sources are needed for video sigmoidoscopes. Halogen or xenon light sources can be used with fiberoptic sigmoidoscopes.
*Cost is $280 when purchased with a sigmoidoscope.

systems require higher quality light sources as well as video processors. Thus, they involve much of the expense of the complete video system without the image quality.

The fundamentals of a fiberoptic sigmoidoscope and proper grasping of the control head are shown in Figure 1.1. On the control head are up-down and left-right control levers. These levers control wires that pass down the shaft of the instrument and bend the distal 10 cm (the "bending section") of the scope. In essentially all the models available, the controls can deflect the tip 180° in both the up and down directions and 160° in both the right and left directions. When the distal tip is deflected maximally in both the up or down

**Table 1.2** *Flexible Video Sigmoidoscopes*

| Manufacturer/Model | Working Length (cm) | Diameter of Insertion Tube (mm) | Working Channel Diameter (mm) | Angle of View | Depth of Field (mm) (Range) | Price |
|---|---|---|---|---|---|---|
| Fujinon ES-300 ER | 79 | 13 | 3.2 | 125° | 5–100 | $10,300 |
| Olympus CF-100S | 63 | 13.3 | 3.2 | 140° | 5–100 | $9980 |
| Pentax ES-3801* | 70 | 12.8 | 3.8 | 120° | 5–100 | $10,300 |

Air and water insufflation are automatic on all models. All models are fully immersible for purposes of disinfection.
*Pentax scopes have a forward water jet for clearing debris off the mucosa.

**Table 1.3** *Electronic Video Processors*

| Manufacturer/Model | Price | Monitor Price Range |
|---|---|---|
| Fujinon EPX-301C | $17,800 | $710–$2150 |
| Olympus CV-100* | $13,400 | $435–$2112 |
| Pentax EPM-3000 | $15,500 | $1275–$2175 |

*Must be accompanied by the CVL-U20 light source at a cost of $9060. In the Fujinon and Pentax systems, the light source is integrated into the processor.

direction and the right or left direction, the bending section will "hairpin," allowing visualization of the instrument shaft (Fig. 1.2). This maneuver is used to examine the very distal rectum for polyps and internal hemorrhoids. Most models have locking levers adjacent to the directional control knobs that will fix the up-down or right-left deflection as desired. Tip deflection should not be attempted unless the locking levers are released to the "free" position. The inlet to the suction channel allows passage of accessories, such as biopsy forceps. Two buttons are located on top of the control head: one allows suction and the other is used for either air or water insufflation. Holding a finger lightly over the button will insufflate air; depressing the button fully insufflates water. The image is viewed through an eyepiece that has a focusing ring. The umbilical cord connects the control head to the light source.

Figure 1.3 shows the distal end of a flexible sigmoidoscope. The air-water nozzle is shaped so that water is directed over the objective lens, clearing it of feces or other adherent material that may obscure the image.

Figure 1.4 shows the internal structure of the distal end of a fiberoptic sigmoidoscope in cross-section. The tips of the fiberoptic and video sigmoidoscopes are similar, except that the objective lens system in a fiberoptic scope overlies a fiberoptic bundle (the image guide bundle) that carries the image directly to the examiner's eye. In the video system the objective lens overlies a television chip (the "charged coupled device" or CCD).

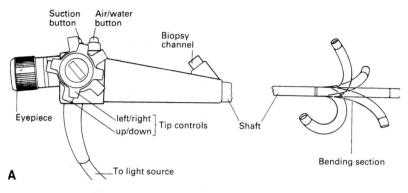

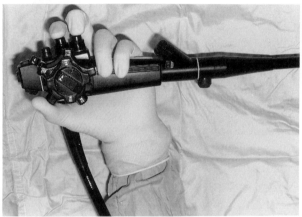

**Fig. 1.1** *(A) The four operating sections of a fiberoptic sigmoidoscope. (Reprinted by permission from Cotton PB, Williams CB. Practical gastrointestinal endoscopy. 3rd ed. Oxford: Blackwell Science, 1990.) (B) Grasping the control head of a video sigmoidoscope. The index finger operates the suction valve and the middle finger operates the air-water valve.*

Figure 1.5 shows the image of a fiberoptic sigmoidoscope as viewed through the eyepiece. The image is circular, and a single black notch is visible on the perimeter. This notch marks the direction in which upward deflection of the bending section will move the visual field; it is sometimes referred to as the "12 o'clock" position in the image. Right, down, and left deflection of the bending section will move the image in the 3, 6, and 9 o'clock positions, respectively.

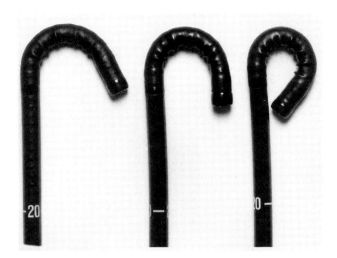

**Fig. 1.2** *Operation of the bending section. The left photograph shows the bending section deflected in the maximum right position (160°) mode. The center photograph shows the bending section in the maximum up position (180°). The right photograph shows both deflections simultaneously; this causes the tip to "hairpin," allowing a view of the insertion tube.*

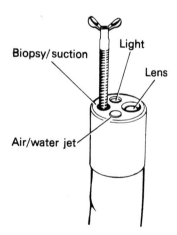

**Fig. 1.3** *The distal tip of a sigmoidoscope. (Reprinted by permission from Cotton PB, Williams CB. Practical gastrointestinal endoscopy. 3rd ed. Oxford: Blackwell Science, 1990.)*

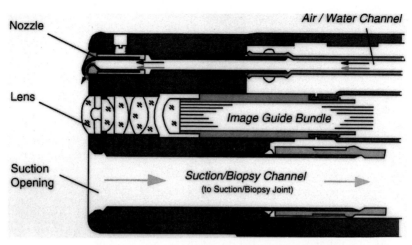

**Fig. 1.4** *Cross-section of the distal tip of a fiberoptic sigmoidoscope. The fiberoptic illumination bundle is not shown. (Courtesy Olympus Corp, Lake Success, NY.)*

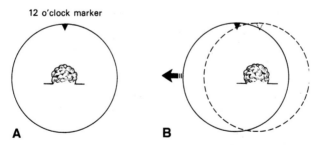

**Fig. 1.5** *(A) Fiberscopes have a marker at the 12 o'clock position. (Reprinted by permission from Cotton PB, Williams CB. Practical gastrointestinal endoscopy. 3rd ed. Oxford: Blackwell Science, 1990.) (B) Deflection of the tip to the left moves the visual field to the 9 o'clock direction. (Reprinted by permission from Cotton PB, Williams CB. Practical gastrointestinal endoscopy. 3rd ed. Oxford: Blackwell Science, 1990.)*

The internal structure of a sigmoidoscope consists of four independent operating systems: 1) a set of pulling wires for deflecting the bending section, 2) a suction system that also allows access for instruments, 3) an air-water insufflation system, and 4) the image system. These features are depicted schematically in Figure 1.6. Under the control head is a separate access for water insufflation (not shown). In Olympus sigmoidoscopes this separate access channel runs down the insertion tube and connects near the bending section to the water insufflation channel as it exits to the air-water nozzle. Thus, this separate access is used occasionally to clear debris impacted in the air-water nozzle. In Fujinon and Pentax instruments, the separate access on the bottom of the control head connects to a channel that exits the distal tip separately from the air-water nozzle. The manufacturers refer to this channel as a "water jet." It is designed to inject water straight out the distal tip, allowing clearing of debris from the mucosa. The mechanical bending system, the air and water insufflation systems, and the suction-biopsy channel system of flexible and video sigmoidoscopes are identical. Likewise, both fiberoptic and video sigmoidoscopes use fiberoptic bundles to transmit light from an external source into the colon.

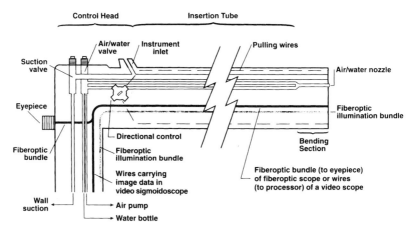

**Fig. 1.6** *Schematic diagram of the internal structure of a sigmoidoscope. The internal operating systems of fiberoptic and video sigmoidoscopes are similar, except for image transmission (see text).*

Image transmission differs fundamentally in fiberoptic and video sigmoidoscopes, as depicted in Figure 1.6. In a fiberoptic scope the image is transmitted via a fiberoptic bundle directly to a lens system in the viewing eyepiece. In a video sigmoidoscope, reflected light from the colon is focused onto light-sensitive picture elements ("pixels") in the CCD. The pixels on the CCD are arranged in a precise grid (Fig. 1.7) and generate an electronic signal that is transmitted by wires through the sigmoidoscope to a video processor. The video processor sorts the pixel data by grid location and converts this electronic data into a signal appropriate for display on a video monitor.

The signal from the CCD chip in all commercially available video sigmoidoscopes is monochromatic (black and white). Color is artificially reproduced by one of two methods. Fujinon and Pentax sigmoidoscopes use red-green-blue sequencing to reproduce color (see Fig. 1.7). In red-green-blue sequencing light from a xenon lamp

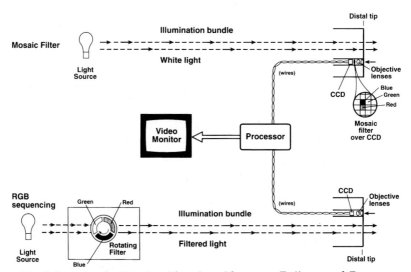

**Fig. 1.7** *Color reproduction in video sigmoidoscopes. Fujinon and Pentax sigmoidoscopes use red-green-blue (RGB) sequencing. Olympus sigmoidoscopes use "color-chip" technology. (Reprinted by permission from Raskin J, Nord J. Colonoscopy. New York: Igaku-Shoin [in press].)*

passes through a spinning disc that sequentially rotates red, green, and blue filters through the light path. The sequences of filtered light pass down the illumination bundles to the colonic lumen, and the reflected images are focused on the CCD chip. The data are sent to the video processor, which analyzes and sorts the sequential images resulting from the color filtered illumination and artificially recreates color in the image transmitted to the monitor.

Olympus endoscopes marketed in the United States reproduce color by a method often referred to as "color-chip" technology. In this method white light is used to illuminate the colon. Reflected light from the colon passes through a mosaic filter before reaching the CCD chip. The mosaic filter consists of a grid of tiny red, green, and blue filters, each of which overlies a single pixel in the CCD in a precise and fixed manner so that each pixel corresponds to a color. The processor sorts the information from the pixels and reproduces color accordingly in the video image (see Fig. 1.7).

### *Optimal Length and Diameter of Flexible Sigmoidoscopes*

The optimal length for flexible sigmoidoscopes is 60 to 70 cm. Thirty-five centimeter scopes cost the same as longer scopes and it may be faster to learn their use. However, the yield of pathologic findings results is 20% to 25% greater with a 60-cm scope compared with a 35-cm scope. To substantially improve the yield of pathologic findings over a 60-cm scope, it is really necessary to use a colonoscopy preparation, a colonoscope, and sedation. Colonoscopy is a procedure requiring much more training than flexible sigmoidoscopy, typically over 100 supervised procedures. Therefore, the optimal length of instrument for the beginner planning a purchase is the 60- to 70-cm instrument.

The diameter of the insertion tube is probably of less importance than length to the purchase decision. Thinner instruments are more flexible and may therefore be more comfortable for the patient as well as less likely to produce perforation when pushed against a fixed area in the sigmoid colon. Thicker instruments, however, may achieve a greater depth of penetration. Most currently available instruments are of comparable insertion tube diameter (Table 1.4).

**Table 1.4** *Fiberoptic Sigmoidoscopes*

| Manufacturer/Model | Working Length (cm) | Diameter of Insertion Tube (mm) | Working Channel Diameter (mm) | Angle of View | Depth of Field (mm) (Range) | Price (U.S.) (6/1/94) |
|---|---|---|---|---|---|---|
| Fujinon | | | | | | |
| SIG-GP | 65 | 11.8 | 3.2 | 105° | 3–100 | $4650 |
| FS7-ER2 | 67 | 13 | 3.2 | 125° | 5–100 | $9800 |
| Olympus | | | | | | |
| OSF-2 | 60 | 12.2 | 3.2 | 100° | 3–100 | $4920 |
| CF-P20S | 63 | 12.2 | 3.2 | 120° | 5–100 | $10,300 |
| Pentax | | | | | | |
| FS-34P2 | 70 | 11.5 | 3.5 | 120° | 3–100 | $4500 |
| FS-38X | 70 | 12.8 | 3.8 | 120° | 3–100 | $10,000 |
| Welch-Allyn | | | | | | |
| FX-100 | 65 | 13.5 | 3.2 | 100° | 3–100 | $4995 |

In general, a large diameter working channel is better. Larger diameter channels allow for faster and more effective suctioning of retained liquid and fecal material. However, for the purpose of routine examination, including passage of biopsy forceps, any channel of 2.8 mm or greater in diameter is adequate.

## Optics

Although there are subjective and objective differences between the images produced by different manufacturers, particularly for video systems, all provide very satisfactory images for clinical use. In general, the resolution of video instruments is greater than that of fiberoptic instruments, except at close range. However, as stated earlier, fiberoptic instruments allow completely adequate examinations. Wider angle of view and greater depth of field penetration (see Table 1.4) are seldom crucial, but may offer some advantage in passing sharp turns and in seeing behind haustral folds and rectal valves.

## Air Insufflation

Some of the more inexpensive commercially available fiberoptic light sources do not include air pumps. In this case air must be injected manually, which few find acceptable. Since air pumps add little to the cost of a light source, it is always preferable to purchase a light source with an air pump.

Sigmoidoscopists should remember that all manufacturers' air pumps will continue to insufflate air at luminal pressures that exceed cecal bursting pressure. Therefore, caution must be exercised during air insufflation. Optimally, a range of air flow rates is available, which includes low rates (<10 mL/sec). Pentax air flow rates tend to be particularly high, on the order of 40 to 55 mL/sec.

## Power and Light Sources

Both fiberoptic and video systems illuminate the bowel via light generated from an external power source and conducted down a noncoherent fiberoptic bundle to one or two exit areas on the distal tip of the sigmoidoscope.

Halogen light sources are low cost (see Table 1.1) and provide adequate light for fiberoptic sigmoidoscopy (Fig. 1.8). In general the quality of photography with halogen light sources is lower. If photography capability is desired, be certain to purchase an appropriate light source. Flash capability of the light source allows quality images and immediate hard copy. All the xenon light sources provide excellent photographic capabilities. Excellent video tape recordings can be made by attaching a VCR to any of the video systems.

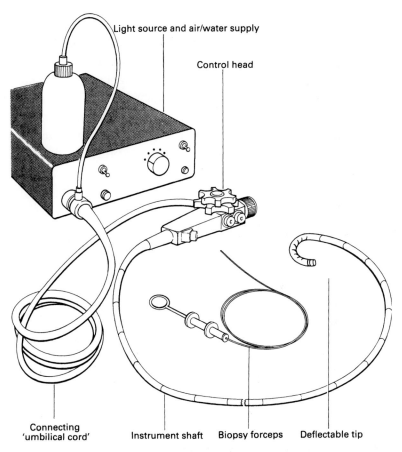

Light source and air/water supply

Control head

Connecting 'umbilical cord'

Instrument shaft     Biopsy forceps     Deflectable tip

**Fig. 1.8** *The simplest (and least expensive) flexible sigmoidoscope system involves a halogen light source and fiberoptic sigmoidoscope. (Reprinted by permission from Cotton PB, Williams CB. Practical gastrointestinal endoscopy. 3rd ed. Oxford: Blackwell Science, 1990.)*

Video systems also allow a range of options for still image production, some of which (such as the mavigraph) involve considerable additional expense.

### Video Processors

To operate a video sigmoidoscope or to use a video converter for a fiberoptic sigmoidoscope, a video processor and light source are needed (Fig. 1.9). In the Fujinon and Pentax systems, the processor and light source are integrated. In the Olympus system, the processor and light source are discrete units. Manufacturers generally make only one video processor for all their video endoscopes, and these machines are expensive (see Table 1.3). The combined cost of the video sigmoidoscope, video processor, light source, video monitor, and a cart generally reaches $30,000+. The addition of components such as a computer, printer, VCR, and mavigraph can raise the cost to over $50,000. This generally provides an immediate explanation for why most primary care office practices still use fiberoptic sigmoidoscopes.

### Video Monitors

Each manufacturer offers several video monitors with a range of price and performance. When purchasing a video system, a critical factor to remember is that the components are arranged in series.

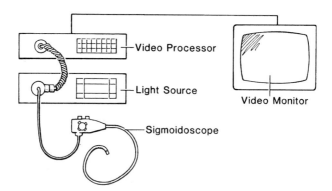

**Fig. 1.9** *Basic elements of a video sigmoidoscope system. In the Pentax and Fujinon systems, the light source and video processor are integrated.*

Therefore, the performance of the system will reflect the performance of the weakest component. For example, a high-performance monitor combined with an older video processor and sigmoidoscope will waste the performance of the monitor. All the components should have comparable performance.

■ ACCESSORIES

Both fiberoptic and video sigmoidoscope systems are best placed on a stable rolling cart (Fig. 1.10). The cart allows mobility of the system between rooms if needed, and can facilitate comfortable positioning and repositioning of the unit during an examination. Accessories,

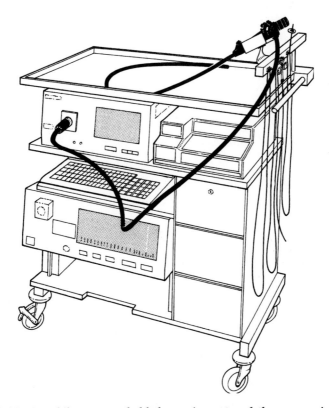

**Fig. 1.10** *A mobile cart can hold the equipment and the accessories. (Reprinted by permission from Cotton PB, Williams CB. Practical gastrointestinal endoscopy. 3rd ed. Oxford: Blackwell Science, 1990.)*

such as gauze pads or wash cloths, gloves, tubes of lubricant jelly, specimen bottles, and report forms, can be stored on the cart shelves or in the drawers that are available in some commercial endoscope carts.

Sigmoidoscopes generally come with a standard set of accessories, including a carrying case, cleaning equipment, extra valves, and, in some cases, biopsy forceps. Endoscope manufacturers make endoscope accessories and several companies specialize in endoscopic accessories. Some companies specialize in making low-cost accessories that generally are acceptable for clinical use. All companies offer disposable cytology brushes (Fig. 1.11) and both reusable and disposable biopsy forceps (Figs. 1.12 and 1.13).

Performance of cold mucosal biopsy material through flexible sigmoidoscopes is a perfectly appropriate procedure for primary

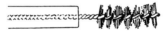

**Fig. 1.11** *Cytology brush with outer sleeve. (Reprinted by permission from Cotton PB, Williams CB. Practical gastrointestinal endoscopy. 3rd ed. Oxford: Blackwell Science, 1990.)*

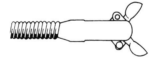

**Fig. 1.12** *Biopsy cups open. (Reprinted by permission from Cotton PB, Williams CB. Practical gastrointestinal endoscopy. 3rd ed. Oxford: Blackwell Science, 1990.)*

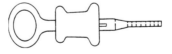

**Fig. 1.13** *Control handle for forceps. (Reprinted by permission from Cotton PB, Williams CB. Practical gastrointestinal endoscopy. 3rd ed. Oxford: Blackwell Science, 1990.)*

care physicians performing flexible sigmoidoscopy. The specimens obtained contain only mucosa and there is essentially no risk of perforation, provided the forceps are not forcibly pushed against the colonic wall. For most purposes any of the commercially available biopsy forceps will provide acceptable specimens for routine use at sigmoidoscopy. In general, the size of biopsy specimens is proportional to the forceps size and they generally are larger when obtained with forceps having fenestrations in the cups (Fig. 1.14). The needle helps fix the forceps on the mucosa and prevent slippage before closure. Alligator forceps are believed to allow better cutting of the tissue, which may reduce bleeding from the biopsy site. Very large "jumbo" forceps require larger channel diameter instruments for passage.

A suction trap (Fig. 1.15) should be available for collecting liquid samples for culture and sensitivity, parasitology, or *Clostridium difficile* antigen or toxin assay.

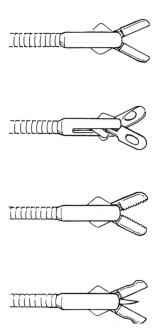

**Fig. 1.14** *Variations in forceps design. From top: standard ovals, fenestrated ovals, alligator forceps, and ovals with needle and fenestrations.*

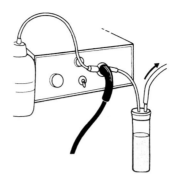

**Fig. 1.15** *A suction trap to collect fluid specimens. (Reprinted by permission from Cotton PB, Williams CB. Practical gastrointestinal endoscopy. 3rd ed. Oxford: Blackwell Science, 1990.)*

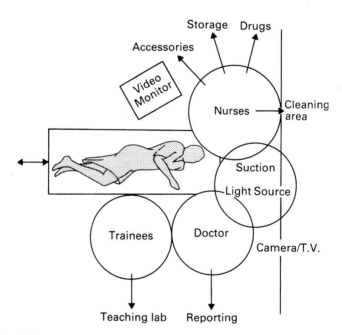

**Fig. 1.16** *Functional planning is important in the endoscopy unit. (Reprinted by permission from Cotton PB, Williams CB. Practical gastrointestinal endoscopy. 3rd ed. Oxford: Blackwell Science, 1990.)*

Special training is required to use polypectomy instruments, such as hot forceps and cautery snares. It must always be kept in mind that if these instruments are used in the setting of an inadequate bowel preparation, there is a risk of explosion. Electrocautery is best reserved for use by the colonoscopist.

## OFFICE NEEDS

A variety of items are useful in the sigmoidoscopy room to make the examination more comfortable for the patient and the examiner. These are listed below.

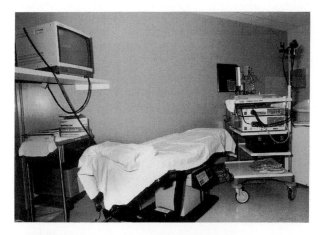

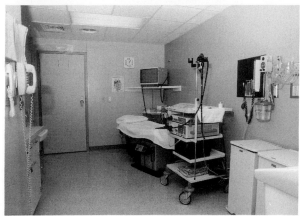

**Fig. 1.17** *Views of a sigmoidoscopy room at Indiana University.*

1. Adjacent toilet with sink
2. Adjacent dressing room (optional)
3. Examination table (hydraulic optional)
4. Dimmer switch on light
5. Rolling adjustable stool
6. Rolling endoscopy cart
7. Storage cabinet for sheets, pillow cases, gloves, lubricant, guaiac cards, endoscope accessories, and examiners' gowns
8. File rack for report forms, consent forms, etc.
9. Cabinet with a lock for hanging the sigmoidoscope
10. Adequate electrical outlets
11. Telephone
12. X-ray view box (optional)
13. Suction apparatus

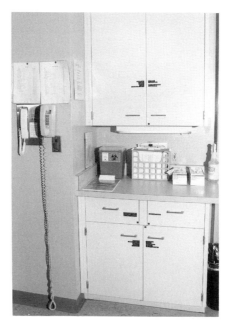

**Fig. 1.18** *Cabinet storage, shelf space, and file rack for forms in the sigmoidoscopy room seen in Fig. 1.17.*

A filing cabinet as well as counter space and a deep sink for cleaning should be in the examination room or an adjacent room. An example of a basic room set-up is given in Figure 1.16. Figures 1.17 and 1.18 show a sigmoidoscopy room set-up at Indiana University.

# Bibliography

▼    ▼    ▼    ▼    ▼    ▼    ▼    ▼

Dubow RA, Katon RM, Benner KG, et al. Short (35-cm) versus long (60-cm) flexible sigmoidoscopy: a comparison of findings and tolerance in asymptomatic screening for colorectal neoplasia. Gastrointest Endosc 1985;31:305–308.

*This is the classic article describing the yield of 35-cm versus 60-cm flexible sigmoidoscopes. The 35-cm scope, although only a bit more than half the length of the 60-cm scope, detects approximately 80% of the neoplasia detected by the longer scope. The reason is that the 60-cm scope tends to bow in the sigmoid colon, which is much less of a problem with the shorter scope. However, since both scopes generally have the same cost, it is preferable to purchase the 60-cm instrument because of the 20% greater yield of neoplasia. If desired, only the first 35 cm need be used during the initial examinations.*

Hawes R, Lehman GA, O'Connor KW, et al. Effect of instrument diameter on the depth of penetration of fiberoptic sigmoidoscopes. Gastrointest Endosc 1988;34:28–31.

*This is the classic study showing that larger diameter of instrument shaft (16 mm vs 12 mm) provides a greater anatomic depth of penetration. The reason once again is likely related to less bowing. However, all the currently available flexible sigmoidoscopes have comparable insertion tube diameters; therefore, this feature is of less importance in choosing a sigmoidoscope.*

Rex DK, Lehman, GA, Hawes RH, et al. Performing screening flexible sigmoidoscopy using colonoscopes: experience in 500 subjects. Gastrointest Endosc 1990;36:486–488.

*More than any other, this study puts to rest the idea that sigmoidoscopes longer than 60 cm are of value for performing screening flexible sigmoidoscopy. In a group of unsedated patients with sigmoidoscopy preparations the authors were unable to pass the scope far beyond the 60-cm mark in most patients. The typical reasons are bowing of the scope in the sigmoid with resultant mesenteric stretching and pain, and, to a lesser extent, poor preparation. Therefore, 60- to 65-cm scopes are adequate for routine flexible sigmoidoscopy.*

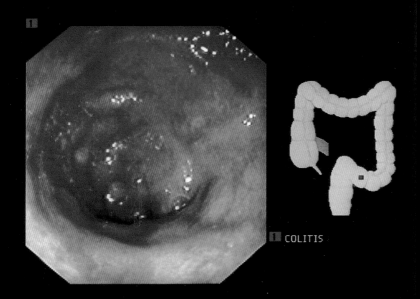

COLITIS

**Plate 1** *Diffuse erythema, granularity and absence of vascular pattern in mild ulcerative colitis.*

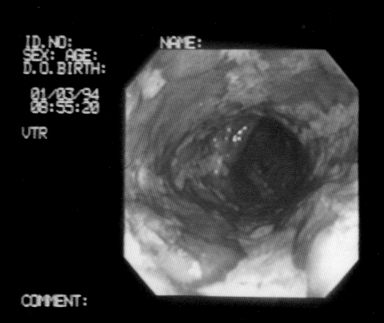

**Plate 2** *Superficial but extensive ulceration with abnormal intervening mucosa in severe ulcerative colitis.*

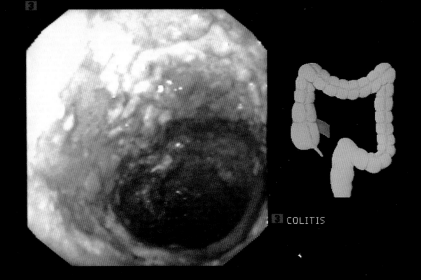

**Plate 3**  *Asymmetric ulceration and cobblestoning in Crohn's colitis.*

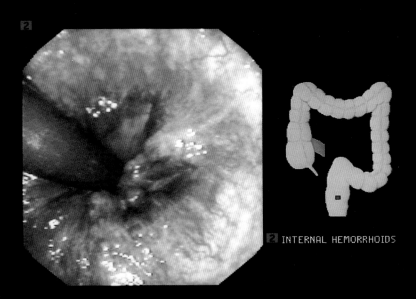

**Plate 4**  *Internal hemorrhoids seen during rectal retroflexion.*

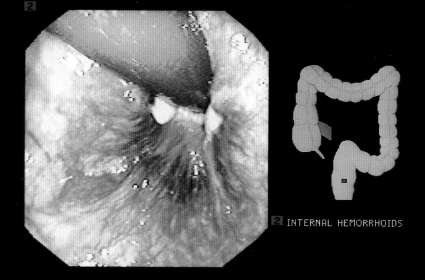

**Plate 5** *Rectal retroflexion showing small internal hemorrhoids and hypertrophied and papillae.*

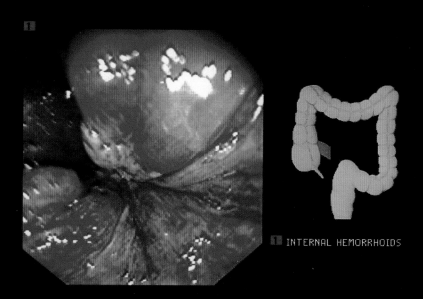

**Plate 6** *Inflamed internal hemorrhoids with bleeding.*

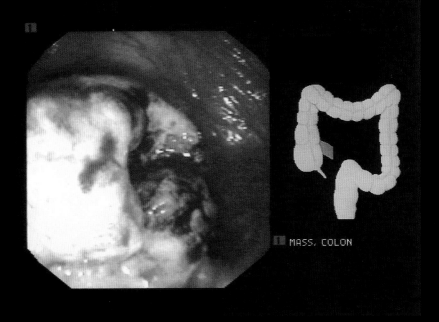

MASS. COLON

**Plate 7** *Polypoid cancer with surface exudate and hemorrhage.*

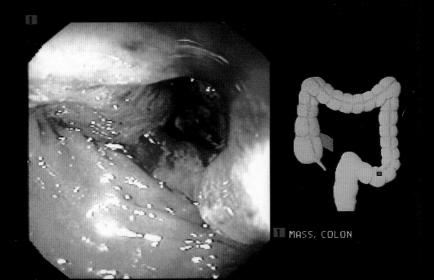

MASS. COLON

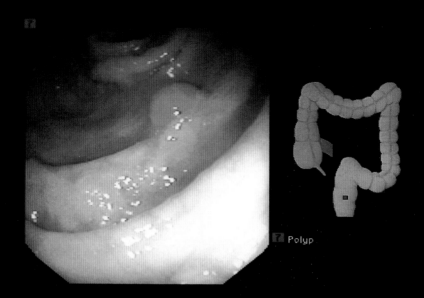

**Plate 9**  *Hyperplastic polyps.*

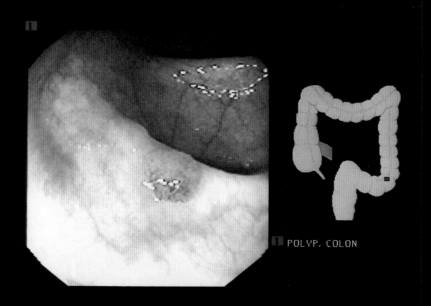

**Plate 10**  *Hyperplastic polyps.*

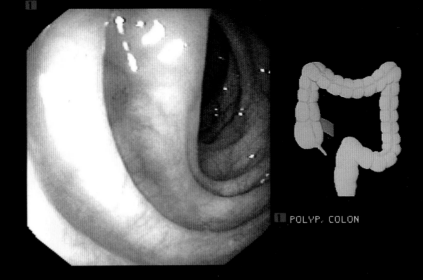

**Plate 11** *Small adenoma between haustral folds.*

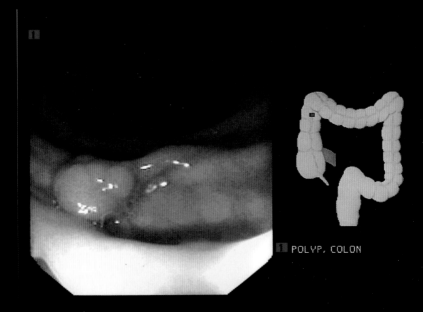

**Plate 12** *Pedunculated adenoma.*

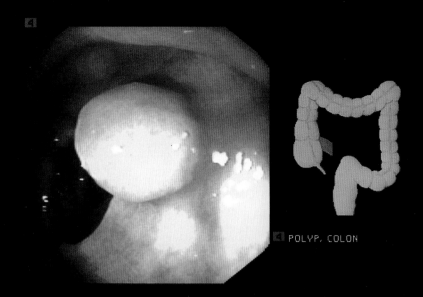

POLYP. COLON

**Plate 13** *Small sessile adenoma.*

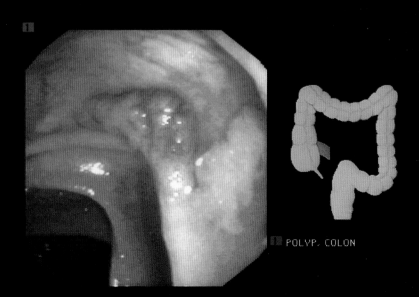

POLYP. COLON

**Plate 14** *"Carpet" adenomas. There is residual mucus adjacent to both polyps.*

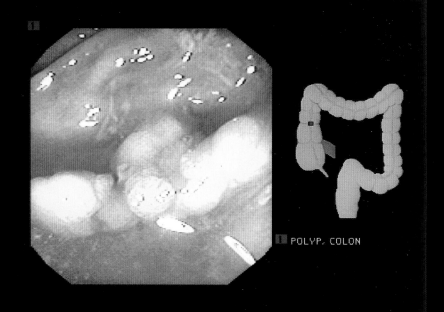

POLYP. COLON

**Plate 15** *"Carpet" adenomas. There is residual mucus adjacent to both polyps.*

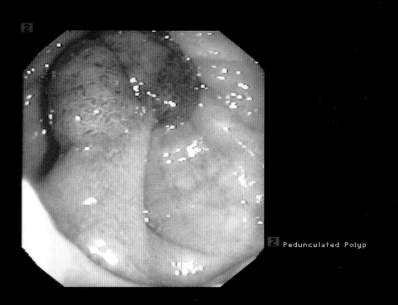

Pedunculated Polyp

**Plate 16** *Large pedunculated adenoma.*

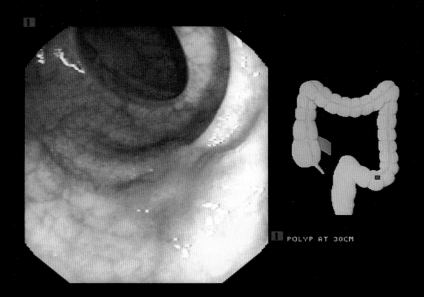

POLYP AT 30CM

**Plate 17** *Large sessile adenoma.*

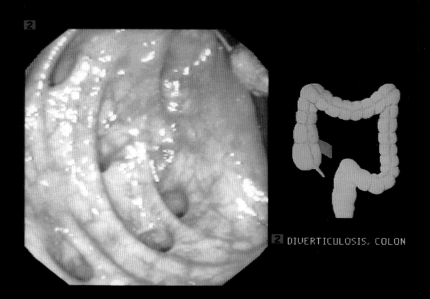

DIVERTICULOSIS, COLON

**Plate 18** *Colonic diverticulosis.*

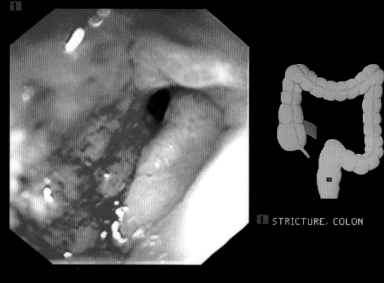

STRICTURE, COLON

**Plate 19** *Benign stricture in Crohn's disease.*

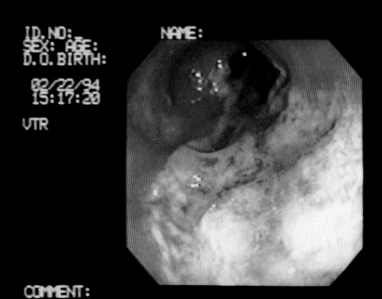

**Plate 20** *Ischemic colitis.*

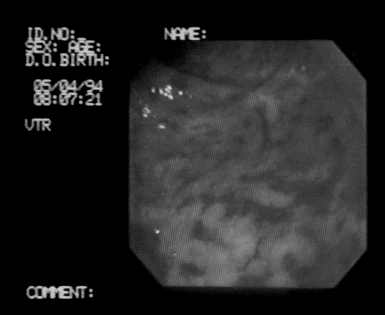

**Plate 21** *Telangiectasias of radiation colitis.*

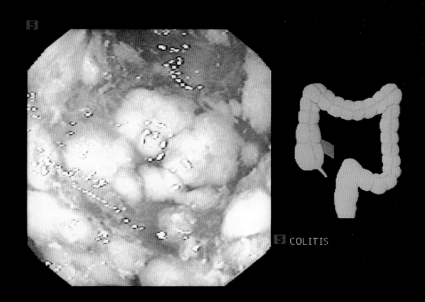

COLITIS

**Plate 22** *Adherent yellow plaques of pseudomembranous colitis.*

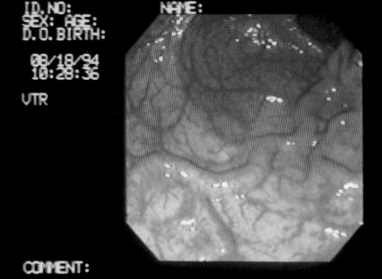

**Plate 23** *Rectal varices. Do not biopsy.*

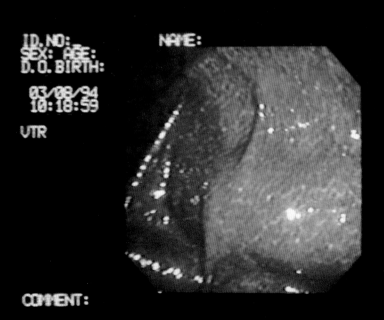

**Plate 24** *Melanosis coli. The dark coloration occurs from depositi[on] of lipofuscin in patients using anthracene (senna, aloe, rhubarb, cascara) cathartics.*

# Patient Selection

▼    ▼    ▼    ▼    ▼    ▼    ▼    ▼

## 2

## ■ INDICATIONS FOR FLEXIBLE SIGMOIDOSCOPY

Flexible sigmoidoscopy either can or should be performed in symptomatic patients who have any of the following symptoms, findings, or indications:

- Rectal bleeding
- Blood mixed with stool
- Blood on toilet paper or dripping from anus
- Acute or chronic diarrhea
- Change in bowel habit or shape
- Assessment of the severity of known ulcerative colitis
- Screening

### Rectal Bleeding

Patients reporting blood only on the toilet paper or blood dripping from the anus after a bowel movement nearly always have an anal source for hemorrhage. Although this type of rectal bleeding nearly always is anal, flexible sigmoidoscopy is still indicated to rule out neoplasm in the rectum and sigmoid colon, and to examine the anus. Patients should be asked about burning or tearing pain during defecation, which is suggestive of an anal fissure. Inquiry also should be made about hemorrhoids, and whether internal hemorrhoids are associated with prolapse.

When blood is mixed with stool, it is more likely that cancer is present. Flexible sigmoidoscopy can be used to evaluate the patient, but if the examination is negative the patient should proceed to full colon imaging.

*Diarrhea*

Diagnosis of the cause of acute bloody, mucoid diarrhea (dysentery) often can be made by stool culture alone. However, a sigmoidoscopy during acute diarrhea may show nonspecific findings of erythema and granularity, which may result from either acute infectious colitis or ulcerative colitis. Performance of mucosal biopsy during flexible sigmoidoscopy biopsy can distinguish acute infectious colitis from ulcerative colitis in this setting, since ulcerative colitis demonstrates chronic changes on histologic examination, even when the clinical presentation is acute (Figs. 2.1 and 2.2).

Flexible sigmoidoscopy is essential in patients with chronic diarrhea. Specific diagnoses, such as ulcerative colitis or Crohn's disease, may be made (Color Plates 1, 2, and 3). Even if the mucosa appears normal, biopsy specimens should be taken, since they may reveal microscopic or collagenous colitis.

*Change in Bowel Habit or Shape*

Patients with rectal cancers may note passage of pencil-thin stools. However, this symptom usually is accompanied by passage of blood into the toilet bowl with the stool. The most common cause of pencil-thin stools is diverticular disease in the sigmoid colon. Changes in bowel habit or shape usually are manifestations of irritable bowel syndrome. However, sigmoidoscopy is appropriate to evaluate these symptoms. Sigmoidoscopy allows the opportunity to rule out the small chance of organic disease, provides reassurance to the patient, and assures the patient that the physician is taking the symptoms seriously.

*Screening*

The other major indication for flexible sigmoidoscopy is as a screening test for colorectal cancer. The rationale for endoscopic screening for colorectal cancer is discussed in Chapter 3. The decision regarding whether to use flexible sigmoidoscopy as the endoscopic screening test for colorectal cancer depends on the initial assessment of risk (Table 2.1). Thus, there are certain conditions for which flexible

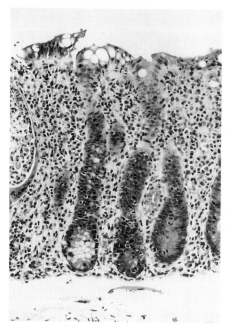

**Fig. 2.1** *The colonic architecture is preserved in acute self-limited colitis. The glands are straight, nonbranching, regular, and extend to the muscularis mucosae. There are neutrophils in the upper third of the lamina propria, glandular, and surface epithelium. In the later stages, as seen here, chronic inflammatory cells may increase in number.*

sigmoidoscopy is inadequate as a screening measure (see Table 2.1). Flexible sigmoidoscopy is primarily indicated as a screening test in individuals with average risk for colorectal cancer. The rationale for selection of endoscopic screening tests is discussed below.

**Familial Polyposis and Gardner's Syndrome:** Familial polyposis and Gardner's syndrome are variants of the same gene defect. They are inherited in an autosomal dominated fashion. Individuals affected with familial polyposis develop thousands of colon polyps beginning in their adolescent years and virtually all have developed colorectal cancer by the age of 50 years. They also are at risk for duodenal adenocarcinomas. Gardner's syndrome bears the same

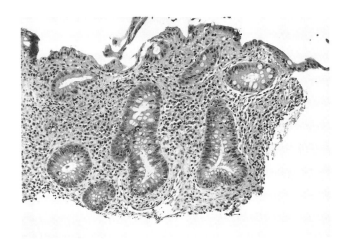

**Fig. 2.2** *Distortion of the colonic architecture is the hallmark of chronic colitis. The glands are irregular in size, shape, and distribution. Branching glands are a common finding. Several glands do not extend to the level of the muscularis mucosae (artifactually removed here).*

risk of colorectal and duodenal cancers, but patients also have tumors at other sites (bone cysts, osteomas, lipomas). The gene defect for familial polyposis and Gardner's syndrome has been mapped to chromosome 5. A number of different mutations in this gene can result in the syndrome. When an affected individual is discovered, his or her blood should be tested by the commercially available assay for familial adenomatous polyposis (FAP) mutations (also called APC for adenomatous polyposic coli mutations). The assay is expensive (approximately $700) and is appropriate only in patients who clinically appear to have FAP or a variant of FAP. The assay is based on detection of truncated FAP gene products that result from mutations that cause stop codons to appear in the gene (Fig. 2.3). The assay is actually positive in only 60% to 70% of FAP kindreds, since not all mutations in the FAP gene result in a truncated protein. If a gene defect in the FAP can be identified, then genetic screening may be performed on blood samples of family members who are at risk. The test is essentially 100% effective in identifying other affected individuals, even though they may not

**Table 2.1** *Selection of Colorectal Cancer Screening Test for Colorectal Cancer and Polyps Based on Risk Assessment*

| Risk Factor | Preferred Screening Measures |
|---|---|
| Extreme risk | |
|   Familial polyposis, Gardner's syndrome | Genetic screening, flexible sigmoidoscopy |
| Lynch syndromes | Colonoscopy |
| High risk | |
|   Ulcerative colitis | Colonoscopy |
|   Positive family history: young or multiple relatives | Colonoscopy |
|   Previous cancer, adenomas | Colonoscopy |
|   Peutz-Jegher | Colonoscopy |
|   Uterine, ovarian cancer | Colonoscopy |
|   Crohn's colitis | Colonoscopy |
|   Breast cancer | Flexible sigmoidoscopy, FOBT |
| Average risk | Flexible sigmoidoscopy, FOBT |

Abbreviation: FOBT, fecal occult blood text.

yet have developed polyps. Testing relatives is less expensive, approximately $200 per person. For probands in whom a gene defect cannot be characterized by the truncation assay, their potentially affected relatives still should be screened by flexible sigmoidoscopy every 6 months beginning in their teenage years. Familial polyposis is believed to account for less than 1% of colorectal cancer cases in United States.

**The Lynch Syndromes:** The Lynch syndromes (I and II) are named for investigator Henry Lynch, who initially described them. They also have been designated hereditary nonpolyposis colorectal cancer (HNPCC; Lynch syndrome 1) and family cancer syndrome (HNPCCII; Lynch syndrome 2). Lynch syndrome 1 is characterized by a predominance of right-sided colon cancers that develop at an

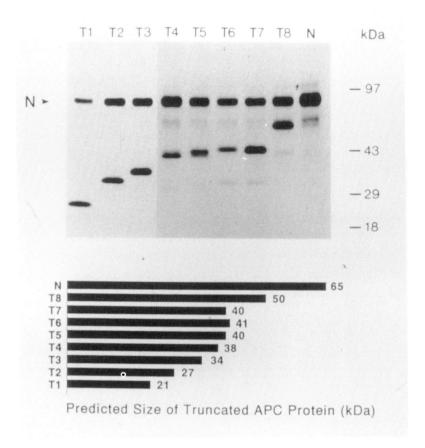

**Fig. 2.3** *Genetic testing for familial polyposis. Most of the kindreds described thus far have nonsense mutations (mutations resulting in stop codons) that result in a shortened or "truncated" protein. The current commercially available assay is based on detection of a truncated protein (thus the term "truncation assay"). DNA is isolated from the patient and used as a template to synthesize the FAP protein. The protein is then run on a gel that separates proteins by molecular weight and is stained. Truncated protein runs faster than normal-sized protein on the gel. The gel in the figure includes samples from different kindreds, each with a different mutation and thus different lengths of truncated protein. The bars below the gel indicate relative length of the proteins. (Reprinted by permission from The New England Journal of Medicine, from Powell SM, et al. Molecular diagnosis of familial adenomatous polyposis. N Engl J Med 1993;329:1982–1987).*

early age (25 to 50 years). Lynch syndrome 2 kindreds have the same pattern of colorectal cancers, but also develop cancers at other sites, including the female genital tract, pancreas, small bowel, and stomach. The term "nonpolyposis colorectal cancer syndrome" is a misnomer, because the cancers arise from adenomas just as they do in other persons.

In every colorectal cancer a careful family history should be taken, with consideration of whether a Lynch syndrome is present. An example of a Lynch syndrome pedigree is shown in Figure 2.4. Clinical criteria for diagnosis of a Lynch syndrome are as follows:

- At least three relatives with colorectal cancer
- One relative diagnosed with colorectal cancer at age <50 years
- Colorectal cancer spanning two or more generations
- One relative must be a first-degree relative (parent or sibling) of the other two

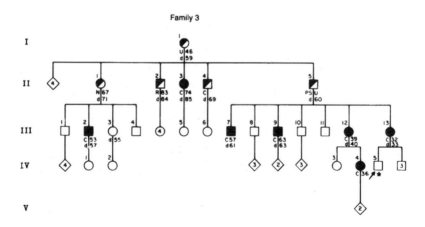

**Fig. 2.4** *A Lynch syndrome 2 kindred. Inheritance is autosomal dominant. C, colon; N, nasopharynx; R, rectum; PSU, primary site unknown; U, uterus. (Reproduced with permission from Archives of Internal Medicine, 1984;144:2209-2211, Copyright © 1994, American Medical Association.)*

Lynch syndrome 2 has the above features, plus cancers arising at other sites (see above).

Together the Lynch syndromes are believed to account for approximately 5% of colorectal cancer cases in the United States. The type of inheritance is autosomal dominant, with a high degree of penetrance in affected individuals. Genetic defects producing the Lynch syndromes are currently being determined. Any of four different genes may account for the syndrome, which may help to explain the relatively high incidence. These genes are important in gene repair, and mutations in the genes lead to failure of DNA mismatch repair. These defects appear to result in mutations in other genes, which in turn cause tumor development. There will soon be a genetic screening test available for evaluation of relatives of affected individuals, although the percentage of kindreds in whom the test will be effective is unknown. When this test becomes available, the results will likely be used to help define the syndrome, and families will be determined to be Lynch kindreds although they do not meet the strict clinical criteria listed above. Because of the right-sided distribution of colorectal cancers in the Lynch syndromes, flexible sigmoidoscopy is inadequate as a screening test. Potentially affected individuals are screened by colonoscopy every 2 to 3 years, beginning at the age of 25 years. Examination using a barium enema also is inadequate, because the adenomas in Lynch syndrome patients are notorious for being relatively flat, and thus difficult to detect by barium enema.

**Ulcerative Colitis:** The extent of increased risk of colorectal cancer in patients with ulcerative colitis is uncertain. Current dogma is that moderate risk develops in patients with ulcerative colitis extending proximal to splenic flexure after 7 years of symptoms. Individuals with disease confined to the left colon do not develop an increased risk until after 15 years of having the disease. Individuals with only ulcerative proctitis have no greater risk than the general population. Flexible sigmoidoscopy is considered inadequate as a screening test for persons with longstanding ulcerative colitis. The current standard of care is annual or biennial colonoscopy with both random and directed biopsies for mucosal dysplasia. However, the effectiveness and cost-effectiveness of such a surveillance program are debatable.

**Positive Family History:** The impact of a positive family history on colorectal cancer is complex. The risk increases as the number of affected individuals with colon cancer or polyps increases and as the age of the affected relatives decreases. If only a single first-degree relative (parent or sibling) has been diagnosed with colorectal cancer, and that individual was over the age of 60 years at the time of diagnosis, there is probably little increased risk. Such persons generally can be screened by flexible sigmoidoscopy. In fact, the American Cancer Society does not distinguish persons with a positive family history from average-risk persons unless the affected relatives were less than 55 years old at the time of diagnosis. In many practices, however, colonoscopy is used to screen individuals with a positive family history of a first-degree relative with colorectal cancer. Colonoscopy is performed beginning at an age 10 to 15 years younger than the youngest affected relative. If negative, it should be repeated at 3- to 5-year intervals.

**Previous Adenomas and Colon Cancer:** Follow-up of individuals whose colons have been cleared of neoplasia by surgery and/or colonoscopy generally involves interval colonoscopy. After a colonoscopy has cleared the colon of adenomatous polyps, most patients can be followed up with another colonoscopy in 3 years. If negative, the next follow-up colonoscopy is performed in 5 years.

**Uterine or Ovarian Cancer:** Women with a personal history of uterine or ovarian cancer may be at some increased risk of developing colorectal cancer. There is no good data on the most cost-effective modality for endoscopic screening of these patients. The choice between colonoscopy and sigmoidoscopy is left to the practitioner.

**Breast Cancer:** Recent studies indicate that patients with breast cancer are not at increased risk of colorectal cancer or of the development of adenomatous polyps. Flexible sigmoidoscopy is an adequate screening measure in women whose only potential risk factor is a personal history of breast cancer.

**Average Risk:** In the United States 5% of individuals reaching the age of 50 years will develop colorectal cancer. Individuals over age 50 with no other recognized risk factor constitute the majority of the population and are said to have average risk. The American Cancer Society recommends flexible sigmoidoscopy every 3 to 5 years. In all likelihood every 5 years is an adequate interval for screening. In the next chapter we will develop the rationale for the use of the flexible sigmoidoscope as a screening test in average-risk persons.

## ▓ SITUATIONS IN WHICH FLEXIBLE SIGMOIDOSCOPY IS INADEQUATE

One of the strongest indications for colonoscopy rather than the combination of flexible sigmoidoscopy and air contrast barium enema is in patients who have positive fecal occult blood tests. If nonrehydrated slides are used, patients with positive fecal occult blood tests have a 5% to 12% chance of having cancer and an approximately 35% chance of having adenomatous polyps. Five large trials of fecal occult blood test screening have examined the sensitivity of double-contrast barium enema and colonoscopy in these patients. All five have shown that examination using double-contrast barium enema missed 25% to 33% of the cancers. In clinical practice, when symptomatic patients are evaluated, barium enema probably is more sensitive, since the tumors in symptomatic patients tend to have later Dukes' stages. However, patients with positive fecal occult blood tests and cancer tend to have early Dukes' stages, making the results of double-contrast barium enema examination more likely to be falsely negative. Therefore, in general, fecal occult blood testing is an indication for colonoscopy rather than flexible sigmoidoscopy alone or flexible sigmoidoscopy plus air contrast barium enema. An exception may be young patients, since the positive predictive value of a fecal occult blood test increases substantially with age. It therefore is probably acceptable to evaluate patients under the age of 50 years who have positive fecal occult blood tests by the combination of flexible sigmoidoscopy and air contrast barium enema. However, patients over the age of 50 years who have positive fecal occult blood tests should be referred initially for colonoscopy.

Iron deficiency anemia is another strong indication for colonoscopy. Particularly in older persons, iron deficiency anemia may be associated with arteriovenous malformations, which are invisible on barium enema examination. Furthermore, particularly if associated with a positive fecal occult blood test, anemia is highly predictive of neoplasia. Because of the need to carefully evaluate the right colon, colonoscopy is preferred over flexible sigmoidoscopy and barium enema for most patients with iron deficiency anemia. Likewise, melena with negative upper endoscopy results should be evaluated by colonoscopy.

## ▍ CONTRAINDICATIONS TO FLEXIBLE SIGMOIDOSCOPY

Flexible sigmoidoscopy should not be performed in a patient who is uncooperative or who is unwilling to give informed consent. Flexible sigmoidoscopy is contraindicated when there is evidence of a perforated viscus. Flexible sigmoidoscopy also is relatively contraindicated in the setting of acute diverticulitis. Acute diverticulitis involves a microperforation of a diverticulum. The perforation usually is well contained by an inflammatory process. However, air insufflation during flexible sigmoidoscopy could theoretically increase intraluminal pressure and perforate the contained inflammatory process. The result would be free intra-abdominal perforation and peritonitis. Although there is little documentation that this complication has occurred with any significant frequency, the theoretical risk of it constitutes a relative contraindication to flexible sigmoidoscopy in the setting of acute diverticulitis. The diagnosis of acute diverticulitis is generally made on clinical grounds alone. Abdominal computed tomography can be useful to rule out the presence of an abscess. If diagnostic uncertainty remains, a barium enema examination usually is the best initial diagnostic tool. The diagnosis is suggested by the results of the barium enema examination when an area of narrowing and bowel wall edema is seen, and is confirmed if a fistula tract is demonstrated.

# Bibliography

▼    ▼    ▼    ▼    ▼    ▼    ▼    ▼

Bernstein CN, Shanahan R, Weinstein WM. Are we telling our patients the truth about surveillance colonoscopy in ulcerative colitis? Lancet 1994;343: 71–74.

> *Like the article by Collins et al, this report casts doubt on the effectiveness of colonoscopy in preventing colorectal cancer deaths in ulcerative colitis. The authors recommend immediate colectomy for all patients with low-grade dysplasia, which differs from previous recommendations. They also suggest that the prophylactic colectomy, the standard of therapy 15 years ago, should be offered to all patients after 20 years of disease.*

Collins RH Jr, Feldman M, Fordtran JS. Colon cancer, dysplasia, and surveillance in patients with ulcerative colitis. N Engl J Med 1987;316:1654–1658.

> *Of all the indications for colonoscopy, surveillance for cancer in ulcerative colitis is the single area where the very efficacy of colonoscopy can be challenged. Approximately 25% of surgical ulcerative colitis colectomy specimens containing cancer have no dysplasia elsewhere in the colon. Over 60 biopsy specimens must be taken from the colon to have a 95% change of detecting the highest grade of dysplasia present. The average colonoscopist takes less than 20 specimens. Many patients with chronic ulcerative colitis refuse to comply with surveillance or are lost to follow-up. Several reports have documented development of colorectal cancer in ulcerative colitis patients in whom surveillance biopsy specimens were negative for dysplasia or who earlier had revealed low-grade dysplasia and then subsequently no additional dysplasia. Patients entering surveillance programs should understand the limitations of colonoscopy in this setting and should still be offered the time-proven alternative of colectomy for prevention of colorectal cancer.*

Elliot MS, et al. Fecal occult blood testing in the detection of colorectal cancer. Br J Surg 1984;71:785–786.

*This and four other studies (see also Frühmorgen et al, Gilbertsen et al, Sontage et al, and Winawer et al [J Natl Cancer Inst]) represent the five clinical trials of fecal occult blood testing in which both barium enema examination and colonoscopy were used in all patients with positive fecal occult blood tests. As is well known, patients with positive fecal occult blood test results tend to have early Dukes' classes. It is remarkable that the range of missed cancers in these studies is 25% to 33%, and is up to 57% for polyps. These studies clearly establish that double-contrast barium enema has inadequate sensitivity for early stage Dukes' cancers and will not be an acceptable screening modality for colorectal cancer. Furthermore, patients with positive fecal occult blood test results, particularly if older than 50 years, should be evaluated by initial colonoscopy.*

Frühmorgen P, et al. Early detection of colorectal carcinoma with a modified guaiac test: a screening examination in 6000 humans. Acta Gastroenterol Belg 1978;41:682–687.

Gilbertsen VA, et al. The earlier detection of colorectal cancers. A preliminary report of the results of the occult blood study. Cancer 1980;455:2899–2901.

Kalra L, Price WR, Jortz BJM, et al. Open access fibre-sigmoidoscopy: a comparative audit of efficacy. BMJ 1988;296:1095–1096.
   *The yield of flexible sigmoidoscopy is compared according to indication. Rectal bleeding has a substantially higher yield for neoplasia than does abdominal pain or altered bowel habit without rectal bleeding.*

Lanspa JJ, Smyrk TC, Lynch HT. The colonoscopist and the Lynch syndromes. Gastrointest Endosc 1990;36:156–158.
   *This paper is a nice review of endoscopic features of the Lynch syndromes. Polyps tend to occur in the right colon and often are only minimally elevated. Screening in Lynch syndrome kindreds is not in the domain of flexible sigmoidoscopy.*

Nicolaides NC, et al. Mutations of two PMS homologues in hereditary nonpolyposis colon cancer. Nature 1994;371:75–80.
   *In this report, the number of genes implicated in hereditary nonpolyposis colon cancer doubled from two to four. This ever-increasing number of genes may explain the relatively high incidence of this disease.*

Powell SM, et al. Molecular diagnosis of familial adenomatous polyposis. N Engl J Med 1993;329:1982–1987.
   *Using a clever assay, the FAP gene could be recognized in family members in*

*87% of affected kindreds. The test could eventually replace sigmoidoscopic screening in kindreds in whom the test will recognize a defect in the proband.*

Rex DK, Sledge GS, Harper PA, et al. Colonic adenomas in asymptomatic women with a history of breast cancer. Am J Gastroenterol 1993;88:2009–2014.

*A recent meta-analysis of epidemiologic studies found that the relative risk of colorectal cancer in women with previous breast cancer was 1.1. The above article reported a screening colonoscopy study in women with a personal history of breast cancer. They were no more likely to have adenomatous polyps than were a group of asymptomatic average-risk control women. Therefore, women with a personal history of breast cancer may have endoscopic screening for colorectal polyps and cancer by flexible sigmoidoscopy.*

Sontag SJ, et al. Fecal occult blood testing for colorectal cancer in Veteran's Administration hospital. Am J Surg 1983;145:89–93.

St John DJB, et al. Cancer risk in relatives of patients with common colorectal cancer. Ann Intern Med 1993;118:785–790.

*Persons with a family history of colorectal cancer were shown to clearly be at an increased lifetime risk. The risk is proportional to the number of affected first-degree relatives and decreasing age at which those affected relatives were diagnosed with colorectal cancer.*

Surawicz C, Belic L. Rectal biopsy helps to distinguish acute self-limiting colitis from idiopathic inflammatory bowel disease. Gastroenterology 1984; 86:104.

*Patients with acute bloody diarrhea and tenesmus can have a nonspecific endoscopic picture at flexible sigmoidoscopy that does not allow differentiation of acute infectious colitis from ulcerative colitis. Therefore, when diffuse, nonspecific colitis is encountered, the endoscopist should take mucosal biopsy specimens. Ulcerative colitis differs from acute infectious colitis. The colonic crypts are shortened, branched, and distorted. Furthermore, extensive infiltration of the mucosa with chronic inflammatory cells and plasma cells is typical of ulcerative colitis. These changes of ulcerative colitis are present histologically even when the clinical presentation is acute.*

Tanaka M, Mazzoleni G, Riddell RH. Distribution of collagenous colitis: utility of flexible sigmoidoscopy. Gut 1992;13:65–70.

*Microscopic colitis and collagenous colitis are part of the same disease spectrum. The patients are typically middle-aged women who present with watery diar-*

*rhea, which may be severe. Endoscopically the colon appears normal. However, biopsy specimens show thickening of the subepithelial collagen layer (collagenous colitis) as well as infiltration of the mucosa with chronic inflammatory cells (microscopic or "lymphocytic" colitis). The subepithelial collagen thickening may only be present in the right colon, and therefore out of the reach of a flexible sigmoidoscope. However, patients with isolated right colonic subepithelial collagen thickening will nearly always have some type of microscopic colitis in the left colon. Therefore, flexible sigmoidoscopy with biopsies of the left colon is a good screening test for collagenous colitis. Random biopsy specimens should always be taken from the left colon during flexible sigmoidoscopy when patients present with chronic watery diarrhea.*

Winawer SJ, et al. Randomized comparison of surveillance intervals after colonoscopic removal of newly diagnosed adenomatous polyps. N Engl J Med 1993;328:901–906.

*Postpolypectomy surveillance generally is in the realm of colonoscopy and not flexible sigmoidoscopy. However, the chance of developing colorectal cancer in the first several years following colonoscopic clearing of adenomas from the colon by an expert colonoscopist is very low. Therefore, after removal of adenomas most patients will not require another colonoscopy for 3 years. If a follow-up colonoscopy is negative for recurrence of adenomas, then the next colonoscopy could likely be prolonged to 5 years.*

Winawer SJ, et al. Screening for colorectal cancer with fecal occult blood testing and sigmoidoscopy. J Natl Cancer Inst 1993;85:1311–1318.

# Screening for Polyps and Cancer

▼ ▼ ▼ ▼ ▼ ▼ ▼ ▼

**3**

## ■ INCIDENCE, SURVIVAL, AND MORTALITY IN COLORECTAL CANCER

Colorectal cancer is the second leading cause of cancer death in the United States, with more than 150,000 new cases and approximately 60,000 deaths from colorectal cancer each year. For those reaching the age of 50 years in the United States, there is a 5% chance of developing colorectal cancer and a 2.5% chance of dying from the disease. If current rates continue, nearly 7,000,000 Americans will die from colorectal cancer. In 1950, the *incidence* (the rate at which new cancers are detected) and *mortality* (the rate at which deaths occur) of colorectal cancer in males and females in the United States were approximately equal. From 1950 until 1985, the incidence of colorectal cancer was increasing steadily in males and decreasing slightly in females. As a result, the incidence of colorectal cancer in the United States is now approximately 1.6 times greater in males than in females (Fig. 3.1) and adenomas are approximately 1.7 times more prevalent in males than in age-matched females. There also are data indicating that the incidence of colorectal cancer is increasing among African-Americans.

*Survival* (the probability of living 5 years after diagnosis) in colorectal cancer has been improving approximately 1% per year over the last three decades in both sexes. Overall, survival has improved 29% since 1950.

The increased incidence of colorectal cancer in males coupled with improved survival resulted in mortality rates for males in the United States that remained steady from 1950 to 1985 (Fig. 3.2). In

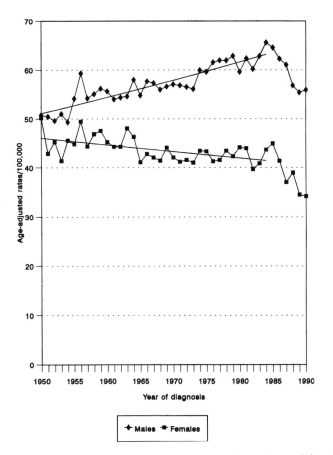

**Fig. 3.1** *Colorectal cancer incidence rates for white males and females in the United States (Connecticut), 1950 through 1990. (Reprinted by permission from Chu K et al. Temporal pattern in colorectal cancer incidence. J Natl Cancer Inst 1994;86:997–1006.)*

females, decreased incidence combined with improved survival resulted in impressive declines in mortality (see Fig. 3.2) Mortality, like incidence, is currently approximately 1.6 times greater in males than in females.

In 1985, the incidence and mortality of colorectal cancer began to decrease sharply in the United States in both males and females. Actually, the incidence of metastatic colorectal cancer began to

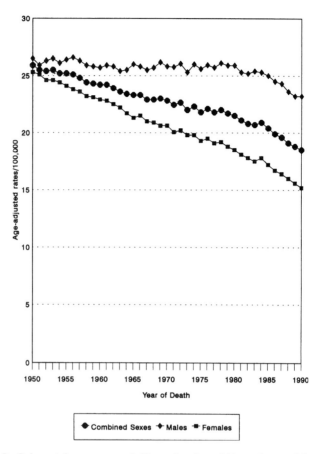

**Fig. 3.2** *Colorectal cancer mortality rates for white males and females in the United States (Connecticut), 1950 through 1990. (Reprinted by permission from Chu K et al. Temporal pattern in colorectal cancer incidence. J Natl Cancer Inst 1994;86:997–1006.)*

decrease in 1975. This was followed by an increase in the incidence of *regional disease* (tumors with lymph node involvement) in the early 1980s and then a decline of these tumors in the late 1980s. *Local disease* (tumors confined to the bowel wall) peaked in incidence in the mid 1980s and then began to decrease. The incidence of carcinoma in situ peaked in the late 1980s and then began to decrease. In a landmark report, Chu et al argued effectively that the stepwise shift in colorectal cancer from metastatic disease to earlier and earlier stages was the result of increasingly widespread application of colonic imaging first to symptomatic and then to progressively more asymptomatic patients. Indeed, Medicare recorded a sharp increase in the number of sigmoidoscopic and colonoscopic examinations beginning in 1985, the year of the discovery of President Reagan's colon cancer. These trends indicate that detection of adenomas at a preneoplastic stage is virtually preventing colorectal cancers.

Thus, it appears we are winning the battle against colorectal cancer! Such trends in incidence and mortality have not taken place in Canada or Great Britain, where there are no established colorectal cancer screening guidelines. In the United States this decrease in mortality has occurred without a nationally organized screening program. Rather, physicians and patients, encouraged by groups such as the American Cancer Society, have developed the system of aggressive evaluation of symptomatic patients, coupled with surveillance and screening, which are widespread in this country. Armed with these encouraging data, we hope you will be further determined to develop expertise in flexible sigmoidoscopy.

## ▓ DETERMINANTS OF MORTALITY

The probability of dying from colorectal cancer is related to the extent of tumor at the time of diagnosis (Table 3.1). This relationship was described by Dukes in 1932, and his pathologic classification of tumor extent is still in use (Fig. 3.3). Dukes' stage A tumors may

**Table 3.1** *Relationship of Dukes' Stage to Survival in Colorectal Cancer*

| Dukes' Stage | Survival Rate |
|---|---|
| A | >90% |
| B | 60–80% |
| C | 40% |
| D | 5% |

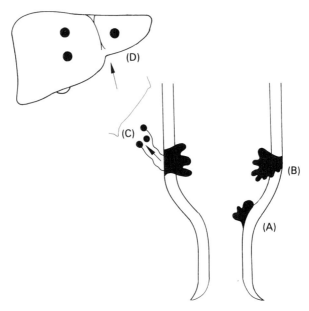

**Fig. 3.3** *Dukes' classification of colorectal cancer: stage A, confined to bowel wall; stage B, involving the serosa; stage C, involving regional lymph nodes; and stage D, distant metastases. (Reprinted by permission from Ellis H, Calne R. Lecture notes on general surgery. 8th ed. Oxford: Blackwell Science, 1993; p. 211.)*

extend into the bowel wall to involve the muscle layer (the muscularis propria) but not beyond. Survival after resection of Dukes' stage A tumors is greater than 90%. Dukes' stage B tumors extend through the muscle layer and involve the serosa. Survival rates after resection are 60% to 80%, depending on the extent of growth beyond the serosa. Classification as a Dukes' stage C tumor indicates that spread to regional lymph nodes has occurred. Survival rates in patients with Dukes' stage C tumors have improved from 30% to approximately 40% as a result of the development of effective adjuvant chemotherapy. Dukes' stage D classification implies distant metastatic disease, usually to the liver, and survival rates are less than 5%.

Approximately 60% of patients with symptomatic colorectal cancer at diagnosis have Dukes' stage C or D tumors. On the other hand, 80% of patients whose cancers are detected at an asymptomatic time have Dukes' stage A or B tumors. Although this has been known for many years, it was not accepted as evidence that early detection prevented colorectal cancer deaths. Factors such as *lead-time bias* (patients with tumors found by screening have longer post-diagnosis survival simply because of earlier discovery) and *length bias* (screening detects a disproportionate number of slow-growing tumors) meant that controlled clinical trials were needed to prove that early detection prevented cancer deaths. Such trials have now been performed (see below) and have proven that detection of cancers with early Dukes' stages and removal of adenomatous polyps prevents colorectal cancer deaths.

## ■ APPROACHES TO PREVENTION

For any cancer, there are several approaches that may be taken to reduce mortality:

- Primary prevention
- Secondary prevention
- Screening and case finding

The optimal approach is *primary prevention,* which refers to the identification and elimination of causative carcinogenic substances from the environment. In addition, identification and reduction of genetic factors important in tumorigenesis is an aspect of primary prevention. Another form of primary prevention is administration of tumor-inhibiting factors. No method of primary prevention is proven effective in colorectal cancer. However, extensive work in this area has implicated several factors that may promote colorectal cancer development and others that likely inhibit initiation of tumor development. These possible associations are the basis of current advice given to patients interested in reducing their risk of developing colorectal cancer:

- Factors that may promote the development of colorectal cancer:
  High fat diet

- Factors that may inhibit the growth or development of colorectal cancer:
  High-fiber diet
  Calcium
  Selenium
  Aspirin; nonsteroidal anti-inflammatory agents

This advice also is generally considered to promote the health of other organ systems.

However, caution should be exercised in advising the ingestion of aspirin or nonsteroidal anti-inflammatory drugs to prevent colorectal cancer. Aspirin has been associated with a decreased incidence of colorectal cancer and a lower risk of metastatic disease. It also appears to prevent the development of adenomas. The mechanism is probably inhibition of prostaglandin synthesis, as prostaglandins are known growth factors for colonic tumors. Despite this, there are significant health risks associated with aspirin, even in low doses. Aspirin causes both gastric and duodenal ulcers, as well as bleeding from other intestinal lesions (e.g., diverticulosis, arteriovenous malformations) that are not themselves induced by aspirin or nonsteroidal anti-inflammatory drugs. Cost-effectiveness analyses have not proven the wisdom of widespread aspirin use for preventing colorectal cancer, and it cannot be recommended for routine use at this time.

A second approach to cancer is *secondary prevention,* which refers to the identification of early cancers that can be surgically cured as well as the identification and removal of malignant precursor lesions. In the case of colorectal cancer, this means the identification of early Dukes' stage tumors as well as adenomatous polyps in symptomatic patients. Flexible sigmoidoscopy can play a role in the evaluation of symptomatic patients, but air contrast barium enema and colonoscopy also have specific indications (see Chapter 2). Adenomatous colon polyps are for the most part asymptomatic lesions. It is paradoxical that when patients present to us with symptoms, we are called on to evaluate them in a fashion that focuses on detection of lesions that could not themselves cause the patients' symptoms. In essence, the desire to identify adenomatous polyps in symptomatic patients means that we are using the patients' symptoms as an excuse to carefully "screen" the colon.

*Screening* is a different approach to cancer prevention. It involves the application of detection techniques for adenomatous polyps and colon cancers in asymptomatic populations. When these techniques are applied to individual patients that we are seeing in the office, the process may be called *case finding*. The rationale for screening and case finding is really the same. In the United States, as stated earlier, there is no nationally organized screening program. Community-based screening programs, largely using fecal occult blood testing, have been sporadically organized. Screening in the United States is therefore performed largely on a case finding basis.

## ■ WHY COLORECTAL CANCER SCREENING WORKS

Colorectal cancer has certain features that make it ideally suited to screening:

- It is a common disease.
- It has serious consequences (death).
- It is slow-growing.
- It arises from a slow-growing benign precursor (adenoma).
- Removal of the precursor prevents cancer development.
- Screening modalities are widely available.

There is extensive knowledge of the natural history of the disease. A large body of evidence suggests that nearly all colorectal cancers arise from a benign neoplastic growth called an "adenomatous polyp" or "adenoma." Adenomatous polyps are extremely common. Figure 3.4 depicts the sequence of proliferative events believed to be associated with development of an adenoma from flat colonic mucosa. Approximately 25% of the population older than 50 years in the United States has one or more adenomas. The prevalence increases with age and male gender. A 70-year-old man is several times more likely than a 50-year-old woman to harbor an adenoma. However, only a minority of adenomatous polyps, perhaps 5% or 10%, ever transform into cancer. For those that do transform into

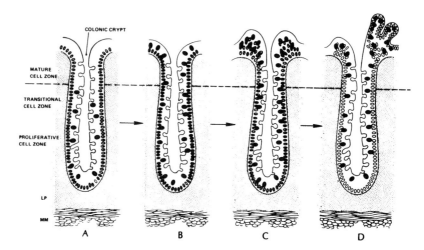

**Fig. 3.4** *Labeling with tritiated thymidine demonstrates the sequence of proliferative events that accounts for development of adenomas. (A) The dark cells illustrate thymidine labeling in normal colonic crypts. As cells move from the proliferative region to the transitional region, cell division is repressed. Cells undergo complete maturation before they reach the mucosal surface. (B) Colonic epithelial cells begin to fail repression of thymidine incorporation into DNA. Proliferation is enhanced. The number of new cells reaching the surface equals the number extruded, and the mucosa remains flat. (C) Multiple cells are present in the surface epithelium that incorporate thymidine. In addition, they have acquired properties that enable them to accumulate in the mucosa, resulting in formation of a polyp. (D) The abnormally proliferating epithelial cells result in development of a progressively larger adenoma. (Reprinted by permission from Lipkin M. Phase 1 and 2 proliferative lesions of colonic epithelial cells in diseases leading to colonic cancer. Cancer 1974;34:878.)*

cancer, the average interval of time to grow and make the initial transformation into cancer is likely to be at least 7 years. The growth and transformation of colonic mucosa into adenomas and then early cancers and then metastatic cancer have been extensively studied, and are now a model for cancer development. The transformation is characterized by a progressive accumulation of somatic mutations (Table 3.2). Accumulation of these mutations undoubtedly determines whether adenomas remain benign or progress to cancer.

**Table 3.2** *Progression of Colorectal Neoplasia by Accumulation of Somatic Mutations*

| Stage of Neoplasia | Somatic Mutation |
|---|---|
| Hyperproliferative mucosa | 5q loss (familial polyposis gene) |
| Early adenoma | DNA hypomethylation |
| Intermediate adenoma | k-*ras* activation |
| Late adenoma | 18q loss (DCC) |
| Cancer | 17q loss (p53) |

Abbreviation: DCC, deleted in colon cancer (loss of this gene also is associated with greater subsequent risk of metastasis).

Unfortunately it is impossible to determine which adenomas are destined to develop sufficient mutations to become cancer. Therefore, it is still necessary to consider all adenomas to have malignant potential. It is clear that identification and removal of adenomatous polyps will virtually prevent the development of colorectal cancer. Once colorectal cancer does develop, it is a relatively slow-growing tumor, probably requiring 1 to 2 years in most patients for the tumor to spread from the mucosa through the bowel wall. This growth pattern of adenomas and cancers provides a long interval to either prevent the development of cancer by removal of adenomas or to identify early cancers and remove them before they have spread to distant sites. Finally, the tests used to screen for colorectal cancer are widely available. All these features make colorectal cancer ideally suited for screening.

The concept that colorectal cancers arise from benign adenomatous polyps is a central one to colorectal cancer screening. The concept generally is referred to as the "adenoma-carcinoma hypothesis." Evidence supporting this hypothesis includes

- Epidemiology of adenomas and cancer is nearly identical.
- Large polyps often have a focus of cancer within them.
- Small cancers sometimes have residual foci of adenomas.

- One third of surgical specimens containing cancer also contain an adenoma.
- Clinical trials show that removal of adenomas prevents the development of cancer.

The adenoma-carcinoma hypothesis is a cornerstone of the rationale for endoscopic screening, since endoscopy is superior to any other method for the detection of adenomatous polyps. For certain high-risk conditions, the best endoscopic screening test is colonoscopy. (Assessment of risk is discussed in detail in Chapter 2.) Flexible sigmoidoscopy is primarily used for screening average-risk persons, who are defined as being 50 years of age or older and having an absence of other recognized risk factors. Average-risk persons comprise approximately 80% of the population. In the remainder of this chapter we will focus on developing the rationale for screening average-risk persons for colon polyps and cancer by flexible sigmoidoscopy. We will review not only the role of flexible sigmoidoscopy, but also that of the fecal occult blood test (Table 3.3).

## ▨ FECAL OCCULT BLOOD TESTING

The most widely accepted fecal occult blood test in western countries is the Hemoccult II Card (SmithKline Diagnostics, San Jose, CA) (Fig. 3.5). Like most commercially available occult blood tests, it is based on the guaiac reaction. Guaiac is a natural compound that is impregnated into filter paper and then enclosed in cardboard. Patients are instructed to collect two portions of their stool on each

**Table 3.3** *American Cancer Society Recommendations for Screening of Asymptomatic People**

| |
| --- |
| Annual fecal blood test beginning at age 50 yr |
| Sigmoidoscopy, preferably flexible, beginning at age 50 yr and at 3- to 5-year intervals |

*The American Cancer Society does not distinguish average-risk persons from those with a positive family history of colorectal cancer unless the affected relatives were younger than 55 years at the time of diagnosis.

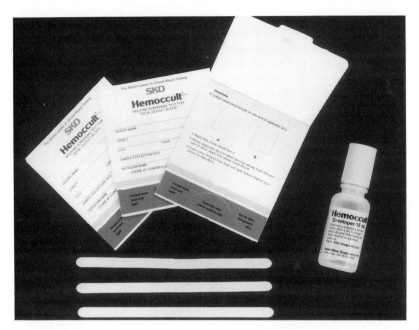

**Fig. 3.5** *The Hemoccult II Card (SmithKline Diagnostics, San Jose, CA) is still the most widely used and best-studied guaiac slide test.*

of 3 consecutive days and to smear them on the filter paper. They then return the smears promptly to their physician or the screening center. At the screening center hydrogen peroxide is added, in the process known as "development" of the cards. A positive reaction depends on the pseudo-peroxidase activity of hemoglobin. If hemoglobin is present, the hydrogen peroxide in the developing solution serves as a catalyst, allowing the pseudo-peroxidase activity of hemoglobin to convert the phenolic compound guaiac to a quinone. The quinone has a blue color, and the color change (which should be unequivocally blue) constitutes a positive test.

It is critical to understand the difference between rehydrated and nonrehydrated guaiac cards. Rehydration refers to the addition of a drop of water to the slide before adding the developing solution. The process increases the sensitivity of the test for the detection of occult blood. It also substantially lowers the positive predictive value (the percentage of patients with positive tests who have cancer or adenoma in the colon). In general, most studies of fecal occult blood testing have not rehydrated the slides and most experts have not recommended rehydration. However, there is only one study in the literature proving that colorectal cancer mortality is decreased by fecal occult blood testing, and in this study the slides were rehydrated. Because rehydration has both significant advantages and disadvantages, it is impossible to make a firm recommendation regarding the advisability of rehydration. In clinical practice, clinicians must consider the known facts and choose whether to practice rehydration.

Most early studies of fecal occult blood testing suggested that the sensitivity for detection of cancers ranged from 50% to 80%. However, these studies often were performed on individuals who already were diagnosed with symptomatic colon cancer, and many had recently had biopsies taken. Thus, they were more likely to have bleeding than persons with asymptomatic cancers. In the past few years it was recognized that the sensitivity of nonrehydrated fecal occult blood tests for asymptomatic cancers is much lower, probably in the range of 30%. Since screening is, of course, performed in asymptomatic populations, this indicates that fecal occult blood testing would have very limited sensitivity in this group. The reason for decreased sensitivity in asymptomatic persons is that they tend to have earlier Dukes' stages, and therefore their tumors are less likely to have the surface ulceration necessary for blood loss. If we recall that approximately half of all persons presenting with symptomatic cancers are cured by surgery (and in some cases by combination with adjuvant chemotherapy), we immediately realize that we must detect two asymptomatic colorectal cancers to prevent one colorectal cancer death. This is because one of the two persons with asymptomatic colorectal cancer would have eventually been cured when they presented with symptoms. If the sensitivity of nonrehydrated slides for cancer in asymptomatic persons is only 30%, this suggests that the expected reduction in colorectal cancer mortality would be only 15%. This dismal number was enough to dampen most experts' enthusiasm regarding the prospects for fecal occult blood testing.

Enthusiasm for fecal occult blood testing was increased in 1993 with publication of results of a randomized prospective trial of fecal occult blood testing in the reduction of colorectal cancer mortality. This study was a landmark paper, and clinicians performing colorectal cancer screening should understand it in some detail. More than 45,000 persons aged 50 to 80 years were randomized into three groups. In one group no fecal occult blood testing was done, in another group annual fecal occult blood testing was performed, and in the third group biennial occult blood testing was performed. It is of tremendous importance that nearly all the slides were rehydrated. The results showed that over a 13-year interval, colorectal cancer mortality was reduced by 33% in the annually screened group compared with the control group. Mortality was reduced by only 6% in the biennially screened group, a difference that did not reach statistical significance.

These results were hailed as proof that annual fecal occult blood testing prevents deaths from colorectal cancer. However, the study is open to several less enthusiastic interpretations. First, there was no reduction in mortality from biennial screening. Many trials of fecal occult blood testing have shown that compliance is poor, and decreases when serial testing is attempted. Thus, one can raise serious questions as to whether the population will comply on a widespread basis with annual fecal occult blood testing. Secondly, rehydration resulted in a very high rate of positive test results (9.8% of all tests performed were positive). This high rate of positive fecal occult blood tests resulted in 38% of the annually screened patients undergoing colonoscopy at some time during the study. Some have questioned the practicality and affordability of a screening test that results in so many persons undergoing an expensive procedure such as colonoscopy. In addition, the positive predictive value for cancer in the study was 2.2%, much lower than the 8% to 12% positive predictive value seen with nonrehydrated slides. These factors combined to make the cost of annual fecal occult blood testing with rehydrated slides very high. Additionally, even if annual fecal occult blood testing were used on a widespread basis, the maximum expected reduction in colorectal cancer mortality would be 33%. A

33% reduction in mortality would still leave colorectal cancer as one of the leading causes of cancer death in the United States. Finally, some experts have argued that approximately half of the 33% mortality reduction in this study actually resulted because so many colonoscopic examinations were performed in patients whose tests were not positive because of bleeding, but because of the rehydration effect. Therefore, this study is open to several interpretations, and in some centers fecal occult blood screening has been discontinued based on the results of the study.

If fecal occult blood testing is used, it is preferable to perform the test on feces passed at home, rather than feces obtained by digital rectal examination in the office. The sensitivity and specificity of fecal occult blood tests obtained by digital rectal examination have not been adequately studied, but there is reason to believe that the specificity in particular is lower than with home testing. As mentioned earlier, clinicians must also decide whether to rehydrate the slides. Nonrehydrated slides have the advantages of better positive predictive value, and diet adjustment during the testing interval is not essential. The disadvantage is lower sensitivity. Rehydrated slides require strict avoidance of red meat for several days prior to and during the testing interval. One of their advantages is improved sensitivity and the disadvantage is lower positive predictive value.

In addition to somewhat meager sensitivity for colorectal cancer, fecal occult blood testing has very poor sensitivity for detection of adenomatous polyps. The sensitivity of endoscopic screening for adenoma detection far exceeds that of fecal occult blood testing (Table 3.4).

### ▧ RATIONALE FOR SCREENING BY FLEXIBLE SIGMOIDOSCOPY

Part of the rationale for screening average-risk persons with flexible sigmoidoscopy is based on the insensitivity of the fecal occult blood test as a sole measure. Thus, many persons with colon cancer and the great majority of persons with adenomatous polyps will have negative fecal occult blood test results. Endoscopic screening is exquisitely sensitive for the detection of adenomatous polyps. Flex-

**Table 3.4** *Hypothetical Yield of Fecal Occult Blood Testing and Flexible Sigmoidoscopy in 1,000 Average-Risk Persons*

| Procedure | No. of Cancers Detected | No. of Persons With Adenomas Detected |
| --- | --- | --- |
| Fecal occult blood test | 2* | 7* |
| Flexible sigmoidoscopy | 2 | 110 |

*Based on 2% of tests positive and positive predictive value of 10% for cancer and 35% for adenomas.

ible sigmoidoscopy with a 60-cm sigmoidoscope will reach on average to the sigmoid descending colon junction. In some patients only the sigmoid colon is reached, and in others the splenic flexure can be reached. Although the region distal to the sigmoid descending junction is less than half the length of the colon, approximately half of colon polyps and cancers arise in this region. Therefore, sigmoidoscopy is not perfect, and colonoscopy in all patients would clearly be more effective. However, colonoscopy is a procedure with greater risk, much greater expense, and a much longer learning curve than flexible sigmoidoscopy. Nearly everyone agrees that flexible sigmoidoscopy is an acceptable compromise between efficacy, cost, and acceptability to patients in the screening of average-risk persons.

The rationale, then, for endoscopic screening is based largely on the adenoma-carcinoma hypothesis. Although occasional cancers are detected by flexible sigmoidoscopy in average-risk persons (approximately 1 per 500 examinations), adenomas are detected in approximately 11% of screened persons aged 50 years and over. As noted earlier, the yield is higher in males than in females and increases sharply with age above 50 years. The first suggestion that endoscopic screening and ultimate polyp removal led to reduction in colorectal cancer mortality came from Gilbertsen in 1974. Gilbertsen followed 18,000 patients with interval rigid proctosigmoidoscopy and adenoma removal from the rectum over a 25-year period. The incidence of rectal cancer was reduced by 85% from expected. Because of some methodologic problems with his study design, Gilbertsen's results were not fully accepted as proof that screening and adenoma removal would prevent cancer. However, two recent case control studies showed 70% to 80% reduction in rectal cancer by proctosigmoidoscopy and adenoma removal from the rectum. There was no protective effect for the colon above the rectum, which was not examined in these patients. In one study the protective effect of adenoma removal lasted for 10 years. The sharp declines in the incidence of rectal cancer and death from rectal cancer in these studies provide the rationale for screening sigmoidoscopy. Because rigid sigmoidoscopy detects only one third of the lesions seen by flexible sigmoidoscopy (Fig. 3.6) and is more uncomfortable and embarrassing for the patient, the current practice is to use flexible sigmoidoscopy.

There is no proof that fecal occult blood testing and flexible sigmoidoscopy have added benefit when performed in the same patient. However, in all likelihood the two screening modalities are complimentary. This is because fecal occult blood testing may have relatively better efficacy for detecting right colon cancers, an area of the colon that cannot be reached by the flexible sigmoidoscope.

## ■ COST-EFFECTIVENESS OF COLON CANCER SCREENING

One model predicted that performing annual fecal occult blood tests on persons over the age of 65 years would cost approximately

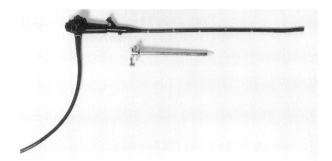

**Fig. 3.6** *The rigid 25-cm proctosigmoidoscope detects only one third the number of polyps and cancers detected by the 60-cm flexible sigmoidoscope. In many cases the rigid sigmoidoscope cannot be inserted beyond 15 cm. Furthermore, it involves more discomfort and embarrassment for the patient.*

$35,000 per life-year saved. In the same model the addition of flexible sigmoidoscopy increased the cost to approximately $45,000 per life-year saved. The National Cancer Institute cost analysis estimated that screening the U.S. population between 50 to 80 years of age with fecal occult blood tests would cost $2 billion in 1994. This cost-effectiveness is approximately $25,000 per life-year saved and is comparable to the cost-effectiveness of breast cancer screening. However, these costs must be offset against the cost associated with colorectal cancer care. Assuming medical costs of $30,000 for non-fatal cases and $100,000 for fatal cases, the annual medical costs of colorectal cancer in the United States are approximately $9 billion. Thus, effective screening for colorectal cancer would have the potential to reduce health care costs by up to $7 billion.

## SUMMARY

In summary, both fecal occult blood testing and flexible sigmoidoscopy are effective methods for reducing colorectal cancer mortality. Whether fecal occult blood testing should be performed with or without rehydration is not certain. Fecal occult blood testing as a single screening measure will fail to detect many colorectal cancers and most adenomatous polyps. Flexible sigmoidoscopy is very effective at detecting both colorectal cancers and adenomas in the distal colon. The optimal interval for flexible sigmoidoscopy screening in average-risk persons is likely at least every 5 years. Fecal occult blood testing and flexible sigmoidoscopy probably are complimentary procedures. Therefore, both screening tests are recommended in average-risk persons. Cost analysis indicated that flexible sigmoidoscopy every 5 years has comparable cost-effectiveness to other widely accepted screening procedures and medical therapies.

# Bibliography

▼    ▼    ▼    ▼    ▼    ▼    ▼    ▼

Chu KC, Tarone RE, Show W-H, et al. Temporal patterns in colorectal cancer. Incidence, survival and mortality from 1950 through 1990. J Natl Cancer Inst 1994;86:997–1006.

*This paper reviews and explains the development of increasing colorectal cancer incidence in males versus females since 1950, and the declines in these parameters in both sexes since 1985.*

Gilbertsen VA. Proctosigmoidoscopy and polypectomy in reducing the incidence of rectal cancer. Cancer 1974;34:936–939.

*This remarkable study was the first to suggest that detection and removal of adenomatous polyps prevented colorectal cancer. However, because of methodologic problems, Gilbertsen's results were not widely accepted.*

Levin B, Murphy GP. Revision in American Cancer Society recommendations for the early detection of colorectal cancer. CA Cancer J Clin 1992;42: 296–299.

*This paper describes the most recent revision of the American Cancer Society guidelines for colorectal cancer screening in asymptomatic persons.*

Mandel JS, Bond JH, Church TR, et al. Reducing mortality from colorectal cancer by screening for fecal occult blood. N Engl J Med 1993;328:1365–1371.

*In this study more than 46,000 adults aged 50 to 80 years were randomized to undergo annual, biennial, or no fecal occult blood testing for colorectal cancer. Slides were rehydrated in 83% of cases. Positive tests occurred in 9.8% of cases. Mortality during 13 years of follow-up was reduced by 33% in the annually screened group and 6% in the biennial group (not statistically significant) compared with the control group. This landmark study proved the efficacy of annual fecal occult blood testing using rehydrated slides and colonoscopy for positive tests. Problems in interpretation of the results are discussed in the text.*

Nelsen DA, Hartley DA, Christianson J, et al. The use of new technologies by rural family physicians. J Fam Pract 1994;38:479–485.

*In a survey of 403 randomly selected family physicians in eight states in the United States, 57% were performing flexible fiberoptic sigmoidoscopy.*

Newcomb PA, Norfleet RG, Storer BE, et al. Screening sigmoidoscopy and colorectal cancer mortality. J Natl Cancer Inst 1992;84:1572–1575.

*This is one of the two case control studies showing that sigmoidoscopy and polyp removal led to a reduction in distal colorectal cancer mortality (see also Selby et al).*

Ransohoff DF, Lang CA. Fecal occult blood screening for colorectal cancer. Is mortality reduced by chance selection for screening colonoscopy? JAMA 1994;271:1011–1013.

*This is a critical analysis of the Minnesota fecal occult blood trial (see Mandel et al). In particular, it was argued that many of the 9.8% positive tests resulted from rehydration rather than bleeding. The authors argued that perhaps half of the 33% mortality reduction resulted from the remarkable number of colonoscopic examinations that were needed, and which resulted in chance detection of adenomas and cancers. The authors believe that fecal occult blood testing is a haphazard method of selecting patients for colonoscopy.*

Rex DK, Lehman GA, Ulbright TM, et al. The yield of a second screening flexible sigmoidoscopy in average-risk persons after one negative examination. Gastroenterology 1994;106:593–595.

*The yield of a second examination at a mean of 3.4 years after an initial negative examination was extremely low. The authors suggested that at least every 5 years would be an adequate interval in average-risk persons.*

Selby JV, Friedman GD, Quesenberry CP, Weiss NS. Effect of occult blood testing on mortality from colorectal cancer. A case control study. Ann Intern Med 1993;118:1–6.

*This is the most widely recognized of the two case control studies showing that sigmoidoscopy and polyp removal would prevent distal colorectal cancer mortality. In this study there was no improvement in colon cancer mortality above the reach of the sigmoidoscope.*

Wagner J. From the Congressional Office of Technology Assessment: costs and effectiveness of colorectal cancer screening in the elderly. JAMA 1990; 264:2732.

*A model for colorectal cancer screening predicted that annual fecal occult blood testing on persons over the age of 55 years would cost approximately $35,000 per life-year saved. The addition of flexible sigmoidoscopy would increase the cost to approximately $42,000 to $45,000 per life-year saved.*

Winawer SJ, et al. Randomized comparison of surveillance intervals after colonoscopic removal of newly diagnosed adenomatous polyps. N Engl J Med 1993;328:901–906.

*This paper provides clear proof that removal of adenomas actually prevents development of colorectal cancer.*

# Preparation

▼  ▼  ▼  ▼  ▼  ▼  ▼  ▼

## 4

**P** REPARATION OF the patient for sigmoidoscopy begins during an office visit at which the need for examination is identified and the procedure is scheduled. The rationale and indication are clearly communicated to the patient. Compliance (i.e., the patient reports for the examination) is dependent on the patient's belief in the need for examination. Physician motivation is an important factor in compliance. Communicating to the patient the need to rule out cancer often is an effective motivator.

The method of bowel cleansing should be described in detail using both verbal and written instructions. The nurse or gastrointestinal assistant may discuss these with the patient. Finally, the physician or assistant discusses the nature of the examination with the patient. The patient is told the position he or she will take during the examination and is given a brief description of the flexible nature of the instrument and how it is guided through the colon. The patient should be told to expect mild pressure during the examination, but that sedation is not needed. Finally, the risks of the procedure are discussed and the patient gives informed consent.

## ■ CONSENT

Flexible sigmoidoscopy is a relatively safe procedure. The risk of a major complication is approximately 1 in 10,000. By comparison, colonoscopy and endoscopic retrograde cholangiopancreatography are 100 times and 300 times more likely to result in a major complication, respectively. Despite this, malpractice lawsuits are filed against physicians for adverse events during flexible sigmoidoscopy at the same rate per procedure performed as for colonoscopy or endoscopic retrograde cholangiopancreatography. The reasons for this problem with malpractice and flexible sigmoidoscopy are not clear, but the problem points out the absolute need for the patient to give informed consent.

During the consent process, emphasis must be placed on the risk of perforation. Bleeding is another risk, but is almost unheard of from diagnostic sigmoidoscopy. If biopsy specimens are taken there is still an extremely low risk of bleeding, unless the patient has a coagulopathy. The reason to emphasize perforation is that it is by far the complication most likely to result in a malpractice suit. The patient should understand that if perforation does occur, surgery will likely be needed to repair it. The other common reason for primary care physicians to be sued is for missing a lesion. Thus, this possibility should be considered a risk of the procedure. We recommend listing four risks on the consent form: 1) perforation, 2) surgery, 3) bleeding, and 4) missing a lesion. Other risks, such as hypotension and respiratory compromise, which are occasionally seen with colonoscopy, are extremely uncommon during flexible sigmoidoscopy, since sedative medication is not routinely used.

Optimally, informed consent is obtained during the visit at which the sigmoidoscopy is scheduled. Obtaining informed consent immediately prior to the procedure is less desirable, since the patient already has been prepared for the examination and may feel less comfortable in refusing.

## ■ BOWEL CLEANSING

The bowel may be prepared for sigmoidoscopy by several methods. Choice of preparation is determined by the information desired by the physician and knowledge of underlying conditions. If there is a known abnormality of the descending colon or splenic flexure, preparation must be good enough to cleanse this region. If a patient has watery diarrhea as the indication for the procedure, then no preparation may be necessary. When preparing the patient for a screening examination, the distal colon should be clean, but it is preferable that the patient not be required to undergo significant expense or effort for preparation.

The majority of patients undergoing routine sigmoidoscopy can be prepared with a simple enema. Using cathartic enemas, such as phosphate enemas (Fleet's), is more effective and less traumatic to the patient than high colonic or tap water enemas. Phosphate enemas are mild mucosal irritants and rapidly lead to evacuation. They may cause mild erythema and occasionally mucosal edema can ensue, altering the appearance of the normal mucosal vascular pattern. Use of other chemicals, such as soap, in the enema fluid can further distort the mucosal appearance and should be avoided. The most commonly used preparation is two disposable phosphate enemas given 30 minutes apart, within 1 hour prior to the examination. To improve the preparation, some physicians have their patients follow a liquid diet the day prior to the examination. Others give their patients a cathartic, such as a bottle of magnesium citrate, in the early evening of the day before the examination. This is particularly advisable if the patient is constipated.

Since one of the goals of flexible sigmoidoscopy is simplicity for the patient, we recommend that preparation for most routine examinations include

- Clear liquids the entire day before the examination
- Nothing by mouth after midnight the evening before the examination
- Two phosphate enemas 30 minutes apart, within 1 hour prior to the examination

This preparation has minimal cost and is associated with less discomfort and inconvenience (Fig. 4.1) for the patient than the use of laxatives. If the patient lives close to the physician's office, preparation at home is preferable.

When placed on a liquid diet, patients should be instructed to avoid red liquids, such as tomato juice and red Jello, since they may alter the colonic effluent and give it the appearance of blood. Remember that diabetic patients generally require adjustment of their insulin regimens when placed on a clear liquid diet. Medica-

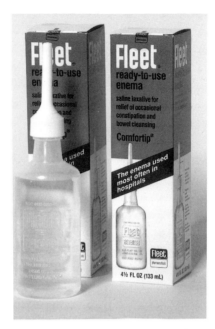

**Fig. 4.1** *Two phosphate enemas on the morning of the examination, accompanied by clear liquids only by mouth on the day before, provide an effective and convenient preparation for flexible sigmoidoscopy.*

tions containing iron should be stopped 1 week prior to examination. The tannic acid in iron causes darkening of the stool and tends to stick to the colonic wall, making cleansing difficult.

Preparations designed for total colonoscopy, such as polyethylene glycol lavage solutions (Golytely or Colyte), should generally be avoided as preparations for sigmoidoscopy. These preparations are excessive for sigmoidoscopy unless a specific lesion needs to be reached high in the left colon.

As stated above, no preparation may be needed when the indication for the procedure is diarrhea. The general rule is that if the patient is passing only water, mucus, and/or blood, without solid stool, then there is probably little need for preparation. If in doubt, a small (<500 mL) tap water enema is preferable to a phosphate enema in patients who may have colitis. Although a standardized preparation is useful, modification for individual patients may be needed. If the examination begins and the preparation is poor, it generally is best to have the assistant administer another enema immediately, then try the procedure again.

## ■ ANTIBIOTIC PROPHYLAXIS

Antibiotic prophylaxis is recommended for certain patients at risk for the development of endocarditis:

Antibiotics indicated:
    Prosthetic heart valve
    Previous endocarditis
    Surgically constructed systemic-pulmonary shunts or conduits
Antibiotics *not* indicated:
    Acquired valvular disease
    Hypertrophic cardiomyopathy
    Mitral valve prolapse with or without regurgitation

The chance of bacteremia during sigmoidoscopy, with or without biopsy, is very low. Endocarditis prophylaxis for flexible sigmoidoscopy is indicated only for "high-risk" valvular lesions. In adults the most commonly encountered high-risk lesion is a prosthetic heart valve. Other high-risk lesions include previous endocarditis and surgically constructed systemic-pulmonary shunts or conduits. Rheumatic valvular dysfunction, hypertrophic cardiomyopathy, and mitral valve prolapse with or without regurgitation do not require prophylaxis for flexible sigmoidoscopy.

When antibiotics are needed for endocarditis prophylaxis prior to flexible sigmoidoscopy, the antibiotics should cover gram-negative aerobes and group D streptococcus (enterococcus). The antibiotics of choice are ampicillin 2 gm plus gentamicin 1.5 mg/kg (not to exceed 80 mg) given intravenously just prior to the examination. The interval of bacteremia, if it does occur, is typically less than 15 minutes, so no additional antibiotics are needed after the examination. In patients allergic to penicillin, vancomycin 1 gm intravenously is substituted for ampicillin.

All recommendations regarding endocarditis prophylaxis and

sigmoidoscopy represent a consensus based on very little data. Thus, they only represent guidelines and physician discretion is appropriate. Endocarditis following endoscopy is rare; there are only four well-documented cases reported in the literature. There is no proof that antibiotics administered before the examination prevent endocarditis. Cases of endocarditis have in fact occurred in nonendoscopic examinations despite appropriate prophylaxis.

There is no consensus regarding prophylactic antibiotics for patients with artificial joints. There is only one reported case of an infected joint following flexible sigmoidoscopy. We do not recommend antibiotics for patients with infected joints. There are certain instances (e.g., artificial joints, breast implants) in which patients may request antibiotic coverage because their physician has instructed them to request prophylaxis for any procedures. Although no data exist to support prophylaxis in these conditions, we recommend honoring the patient's request in these instances.

# Bibliography

▼ ▼ ▼ ▼ ▼ ▼ ▼ ▼

Dajani AS, Bisno AL, Chung KJ, et al. Prevention of bacterial endocarditis. JAMA 1990;264:2919–2922.

*This paper is the basis of our recommendation regarding antibiotic prophylaxis.*

Gerstenberger PD, Plumeri PA. Malpractice claims in gastrointestinal endoscopy: analysis of an insurance industry data base. Gastrointest Endosc 1993; 39:132–138.

*Although considered to be much safer, flexible sigmoidoscopy resulted in a malpractice suit rate per procedure performed that was equal to colonoscopy. The reasons for this are unclear, but emphasize the need to obtain informed consent. The most important risks are associated with perforation and with missing a diagnosis, not only in the gastrointestinal tract, but in other organs (for example, cancer of the female genital tract).*

Hocutt JE Jr, Jaffe R, Owens G, Walters D. Flexible fiberoptic sigmoidoscopy in family medicine. Am Fam Physician 1984;29:131–138.

*This and the paper by Weiss and Watkins describe the experience with bowel preparation in two family physicians' offices. Weiss and Watkins compared one to two Fleet enemas in a nonrandomized, nonblinded study using a 35-cm flexible sigmoidoscope. They found that one enema 1 hour before the examination was as good as one enema 3 hours before the examination and a second enema 1 hour before the examination. Hocutt et al instructed their patients to take the number of enemas necessary to provide a clear return. The papers are included to show that a variety of different preparation instructions have been found to be successful for flexible sigmoidoscopy.*

Holt WS. Factors affecting compliance with screening sigmoidoscopy. J Fam Pract 1991;32:585–589.

*Physician motivation was shown to be a major determinant in compliance rates with screening sigmoidoscopy.*

Petravage J, Swedberg J. Patient response to sigmoidoscopy recommendation via mailed reminders. J Fam Pract 1988;27:387–389.

*A survey of patients over the age of 50 years determined that only 13% who were advised to undergo a screening sigmoidoscopy wanted to receive the test. Common reasons for declining the tests were cost (31%), discomfort (12%), and fear (9%).*

Triesenberg SN, Clark NM, Kauffman CA. Group B streptococcal prosthetic joint infection following sigmoidoscopy. Clin Infect Dis 1992;15:374–375.

*This is the only case report of which we are aware in which flexible sigmoidoscopy resulted in an infected prosthetic joint. No formal recommendations have been made regarding prophylactic antibiotics for prosthetic joints before flexible sigmoidoscopy. We recommend that they not be given, unless the patient requests them based on advice from another physician.*

Weiss B, Watkins S. Bowel preparation for flexible sigmoidoscopy. J Fam Pract 1985;21:285–287.

# Evaluation and Examination of the Anorectum

▼   ▼   ▼   ▼   ▼   ▼   ▼   ▼

**P**RIOR TO flexible sigmoidoscopy the examiner always visually inspects the anus and perineum and then performs a digital examination of the anal canal and rectum. The indication for flexible sigmoidoscopy often is an anorectal symptom. Thus, rectal bleeding may require evaluation of the rectum and distal colon by sigmoidoscopy to rule out colitis and neoplasia, but the examination will most often reveal hemorrhoids. Because of the high prevalence of anorectal findings in the population undergoing flexible sigmoidoscopy, it behooves the examiner to become expert in anorectal disease. This chapter reviews the normal anatomy of the anorectum, the method of examination of the anorectum, and its abnormal findings.

## ■ NORMAL ANATOMY

The anal canal is 3 to 4 cm long in adults. The proximal half is lined by columnar epithelium, and the distal half is lined by squamous epithelium that is modified in its proximal portions so that it lacks normal skin appendages, such as hair follicles, sweat glands, or sebaceous glands. The junction of columnar and squamous epithelium is the dentate or pectinate line (Fig. 5.1). The mucosa and skin form longitudinal folds at this point, termed "anal valves." Visual inspection of the anal canal through an anoscope or with a slowly withdrawn flexible instrument demonstrates the dentate or pectinate line by a sharp transition between the pink columnar mucosa of the rectum and the pearly white or pigmented (depending on the patient's race) modified squamous epithelium of the anal canal. It

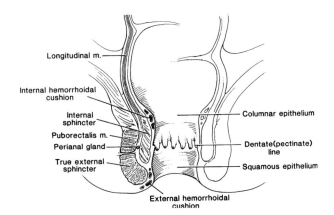

**Fig. 5.1** *Normal anatomy of the anorectum.*

can be easily seen with the flexible sigmoidoscope retroflexed in the rectum. The pectinate line also separates the zones of visceral from somatic innervation. Thus, mucosal biopsies or therapies applied above this line are generally associated with little pain, whereas procedures applied below the line require anesthesia.

With retroversion of the flexible instrument in the rectum, mucosal folds may be seen radiating to the dentate line. These folds, sometimes called the "columns of Morgagni," represent the converging terminal branches of the superior hemorrhoidal artery. The anorectal glands, which produce lubricating mucus for the anal canal, empty at the dentate line. The crypts are the typical origination site for the formation of a perirectal fistula.

The epithelial lining of the anal canal is surrounded by a group of muscles that collectively form the anal sphincter. The innermost muscle is the internal anal sphincter, a circular smooth muscle that lines the upper two thirds of the canal. Anatomically, the internal sphincter is an extension of the longitudinal muscle layer of the rectum (see Fig 5.1). The internal sphincter is not under voluntary control. During rest, the internal sphincter provides approximately 70% of the "tone" or resting pressure in the anal canal. The internal sphincter relaxes in response to rectal distention. This involuntary response is called the "rectosphincteric reflex" (Fig. 5.2). Relaxation

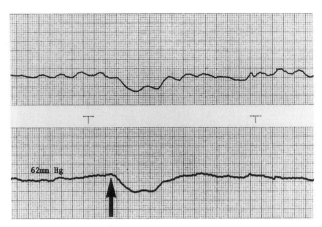

**Fig. 5.2** *The rectosphincteric reflex. Baseline pressure in the anal canal is 62 mm Hg in the bottom lead and approximately 40 mm Hg in the top lead. With distention of the rectum (arrow), the anal canal (internal sphincter) relaxes.*

of the internal sphincter during rectal distention allows rectal contents to reach the upper portion of the anal canal. There specialized sensory receptors have the remarkable ability to distinguish gas from liquid from solid, a distinction that rapidly reaches consciousness. This information is helpful in deciding whether to voluntarily resist passage of rectal contents until a socially acceptable location is found, or to proceed with emptying rectal contents.

Surrounding the internal sphincter is a group of striated muscles collectively called the "external sphincter." Unlike other striated muscles in the body, the external anal sphincter (like the urethral sphincter) exhibits tonic contractile activity at rest. When we squeeze the pelvic floor (as in trying to hold onto a loose bowel movement), the activity in the external sphincter increases and anal canal pressure increases, helping to retain the bowel movement until we can reach the bathroom. On the other hand, when we strain to defecate, the tonic contractile activity in the external sphincter is inhibited. This results in relaxation of the external sphincter complex and a decrease in anal canal pressure, facilitating defecation. For practical purposes, it is useful to understand two of the individual muscles in the external sphincter complex: the true external sphincter muscle and the puborectalis muscle (see Fig. 5.1). The true external sphincter muscle is the distal-most portion of the external sphincter complex. You can see this muscle during visual inspection of the anus. The "puckered" appearance of the anus when the patient is asked to squeeze is caused by the contraction of the true external sphincter muscle. Like all striated muscles, the true external sphincter has a bony attachment. Both ends of the muscle are attached posteriorly to the coccyx, and the muscle loops anteriorly around the anal canal. Thus, when the true external sphincter contracts, it pulls the lower portion of the anal canal posteriorly.

The puborectalis muscle is the proximal or upper-most portion of the external sphincter complex. It is a powerful muscle, and most experts believe it is a very important component of the continence mechanism. The muscle loops posteriorly around the upper end of the anal canal and both ends attach anteriorly to the symphysis pubis (Fig. 5.3A). When the external sphincter complex contracts, the shortened puborectalis pulls the upper portion of the anal canal anteriorly (Fig. 5.3B). When the sphincter complex relaxes during defecation, the puborectalis lengthens and the upper portion of the anal canal moves posteriorly (Fig. 5.3C). You cannot see the puborectalis muscle, but you can easily feel it during the digital rectal examination. With the index finger fully inserted in the anal canal, the finger is directed posteriorly. The palpating finger will detect a

---

**Fig. 5.3** *(A) The puborectalis muscle ends are both attached to the symphysis pubis, and the muscle loops posteriorly around the proximal end of the anal canal. The intersection of the axis of the anal canal and the posterior wall of the rectum form the anorectal angle. (B) Squeezing the pelvic floor to retain a bowel movement results in contraction and shortening of the puborectalis muscle. The anorectal angle becomes more acute. A finger inserted into the rectum and directed posteriorly over the proximal end of the anal canal can palpate the ridge formed by the contracting puborectalis muscle during squeeze. (C) With straining to defecate, the puborectalis muscle relaxes and lengthens. The anorectal angle becomes more obtuse, facilitating passage of rectal contents.*

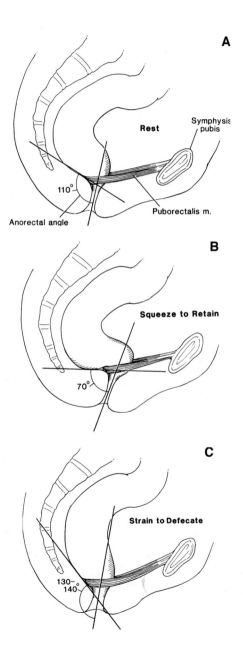

smooth ridge posteriorly at the upper end of the anal canal. This is the sling of the puborectalis muscle. Ask the patient to squeeze and the ridge becomes firm and sharp, and moves anteriorly and up toward the curved finger as the muscle contracts (see Fig. 5.3B). Ask the patient to strain (as if passing a bowel movement) and the ridge disappears as the muscle relaxes (see Fig. 5.3C).

The true external sphincter and puborectalis muscles are part of a group of striated muscles in the pelvic floor called the "levator ani." Although under voluntary control, the individual muscular components of the levator ani cannot be operated independently. Thus, they contract or relax as a unit. As noted above, these muscles relax during defecation. This relaxation is accompanied by 1 to 2 cm of inferior movement of the levator complex. This normal movement is sometimes called "perineal descent," and it can be easily observed during visual inspection of the perineum while asking the patient to strain. The concept is a clinically useful one, since some women develop excessive perineal descent during defecation, resulting in the "descending perineum syndrome." On inspection the perineum appears to balloon out toward the examiner during straining (Fig. 5.4). Descending perineum syndrome is associated with laxity of the levator complex. It often is associated with multiparity, and

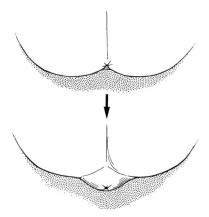

**Fig. 5.4** *Descending perineum syndrome seen at rest (top) and with straining (bottom).*

there may be an associated rectocele, cystocele, or enterocele. Constipation may result because the fecal bolus in the rectum drops so low that abdominal pressure can no longer effectively help to eliminate the bolus from the rectum. Incontinence also is associated with this syndrome and is thought to result from chronic stretching of the pudendal nerves during the exaggerated descent, resulting in eventual denervation of the sphincter muscles.

Notice that the axis of the anal canal and the axis of the rectum form an angle that becomes more acute during squeezing and obtuse during straining (see Fig. 5.3). These changes in the anorectal angle are directly related to contraction and relaxation of the puborectalis muscle. The anorectal angle itself was thought for many decades to be an important factor in maintaining continence. It was believed that an acute angle allowed the anterior wall of the rectum to fall over the anus, promoting continence. This idea has been disproved, but the anorectal angle and how it changes during continence are worth understanding, as they are still discussed.

At the upper and lower ends of the anal canal are normal vascular structures sometimes called the "internal" and "external" hemorrhoidal cushions (see Fig. 5.1). Chronic straining during bowel movements can cause these vascular cushions to enlarge and disengage from their underlying connective tissue, with resultant clinical hemorrhoids (Color Plates 4, 5, and 6). Grading internal hemorrhoids by prolapse is useful in directing therapy. Conservative therapy and simple therapies like rubber band ligation, infrared coagulation (Fig. 5.5), bipolar cautery, or injection therapy can be used for grade 1 and 2 and some grade 3 internal hemorrhoids (Table 5.1). Some of these therapies, particularly infrared coagulation and bipolar cautery, may be applied by primary care physicians. Surgical therapy is needed for some grade 3 and all grade 4 hemorrhoids.

## ▨ EXPECTATION OF FINDINGS BASED ON SYMPTOMS

As with many areas of medicine, examination findings of the anorectum often can be anticipated based on a careful history. Discussed

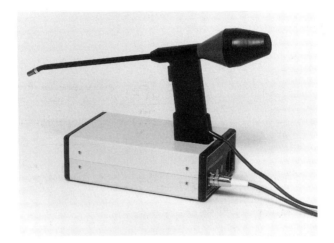

**Fig. 5.5** *The infrared coagulation device (Redfield Corp, Montvale, NJ).*

below are anorectal symptoms that the patient may report, along with their likely significance.

*Rectal Bleeding*

Small amounts of blood on the toilet paper, dripping from the anus after a bowel movement, or passed without a bowel movement are suggestive of an anal source, such as hemorrhoids or fissure. Blood mixed with or streaked on stool is more predictive of a colonic source and is worrisome for cancer. However, there is overlap between these presentations (some patients with anal type bleeding

**Table 5.1** *Grading System for Internal Hemorrhoids Based on Prolapse*

| Grade | Degree of Prolapse |
|-------|--------------------|
| 1 | None |
| 2 | Prolapse but spontaneous reduction |
| 3 | Prolapse requires manual reduction |
| 4 | Irreducible prolapse; may be thrombosis and gangrene |

have colon tumors), and thus a need for colonic evaluation in all patients with recent onset of rectal bleeding.

## Anal Pain with Defecation

Patients with or without rectal bleeding who report a burning or tearing sensation in the anus with bowel movements usually have an anal canal fissure. The pathogenesis typically involves a tear in the anal canal after a hard bowel movement. Part of the pain results from secondary involuntary spasm of anal canal muscles. Examination will reveal the fissure, tenderness in the anal canal, and sometimes a tight anal canal, reflecting high anal canal pressures. Retroflexion of the flexible sigmoidoscope in the rectum may demonstrate hypertrophy of the anal valve in the area proximal to the fissure. This is the genesis of the "hypertrophied anal papillae" (see Color Plate 5). The fissure also is frequently accompanied by an external tag (Fig. 5.6).

## Continuous Anal Pain

New onset of severe anal or perirectal pain should suggest either a thrombosed external hemorrhoid or a perirectal abscess (particularly if accompanied by fever). A thrombosed hemorrhoid will be obvious on inspection of the anus, appearing as a tense, purple, grapelike mass at the external verge that is tender to palpation (Fig. 5.7).

The patient with a perirectal abscess may report drainage of pus on underclothing from spontaneous rupture of the abscess. Coexistent abdominal pain or diarrhea suggests Crohn's disease. Examination will detect exquisite localized tenderness (and sometimes erythema and swelling) in the perineum (Fig. 5.8) or may demonstrate tenderness in the anal canal. Fluctuance is diagnostic but may be absent, as abscesses may be located at a considerable distance from the perianal skin (Fig. 5.9). A fistula orifice may be evident on the perianal skin if there has been spontaneous drainage. Immediate referral to a surgeon is indicated.

Anal pain associated with discharge of purulent material should suggest a fistula (Fig. 5.10) that may be associated with an abscess. The course of fistulae can be predicted by Goodsall's rule (Fig. 5.11).

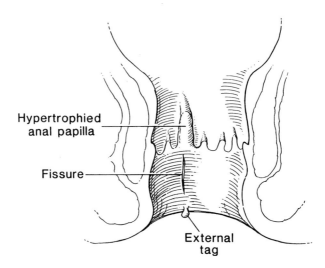

**Fig. 5.6** *The triad of anal fissure, including the external tag and hyper-trophied anal papilla.*

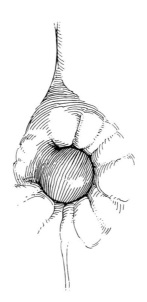

**Fig. 5.7** *A thrombosed external hemorrhoid. (Reprinted by permission from Dunn D, Rawlinson N. Surgical diagnosis and management: a guide to surgical care. 2nd ed. Oxford: Blackwell Science, 1991.)*

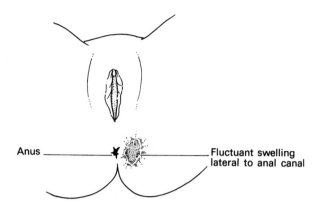

Anus ─────────── ✗ ──────────── Fluctuant swelling
                                  lateral to anal canal

**Fig. 5.8** *The presentation of perirectal abscess. (Reprinted by permission from Bevan PG, Donovan IA. Handbook of general surgery. Oxford: Blackwell Science, 1992.)*

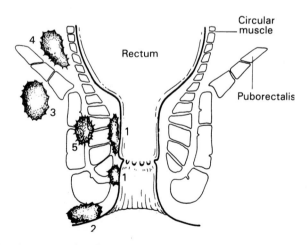

**Fig. 5.9** *Abscesses related to the anal canal: 1, submucous; 2, perianal; 3, ischiorectal; 4, pelvirectal; and 5, intersphincteric. (Reprinted by permission from Bevan PG, Donovan IA. Handbook of general surgery. Oxford: Blackwell Science, 1992.)*

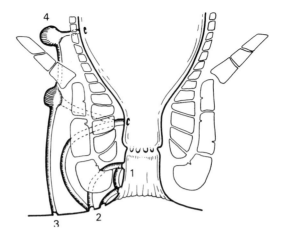

**Fig. 5.10** *Anal fistulae: 1, submucous-subcutaneous; 2, anorectal (low and high); 3, ischiorectal; and 4, pelvirectal. (Reprinted by permission from Bevan PG, Donovan IA. Handbook of general surgery. Oxford: Blackwell Science, 1992.)*

Treatment of a fistula often is surgical, although excision implies a risk of fecal incontinence. Exact preoperative definition of the fistula tract is essential to predict this risk. Medical therapy is adequate in some patients, and particularly advantageous in Crohn's fistulae.

### Pruritus

The simplest etiology for pruritus is poor hygiene. In some cases inspection reveals external hemorrhoids or tags that impede perfect

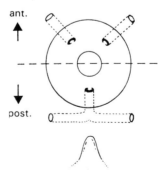

**Fig. 5.11** *Goodsall's rule for anal fistulae.*

cleansing after bowel movements. In others there may be anal canal weakness or deformity leading to small amounts of feces that leak onto the perineal skin after bowel movements. Some persons with apparently normal sphincter strength appear to leave a small residual of feces in their anal canal during and after bowel movements. After wiping the anal canal, motor activity pushes the stool onto the perianal skin, with resulting irritation and pruritus. Vaginal discharges also may cause pruritus ani.

Pruritus ani also may be seen in some serious conditions, such as viral infections (herpes, condyloma, cytomegalovirus) or syphilis. Neoplasms, such as squamous cell or cloacogenic carcinoma of the anus, may present with pruritus. Therefore, careful inspection of the anus and perineum for such lesions is essential. Inspection also should focus on secondary fungal infection of the perianal skin, which will respond to topical therapy. Digital examination should focus on deformity of the anal canal and anal sphincter strength. Therapy usually involves meticulous attention to cleanliness (Table 5.2).

### Incontinence

Many types of fecal incontinence can be successfully managed by primary care physicians. All patients with diarrhea should be questioned about incontinence, since embarrassment may lead the patient to report diarrhea when the real problem is incontinence. Flexible sigmoidoscopy is indicated to rule out colon tumors, colitis, and rectal ulceration.

Initial questioning should include an attempt to determine the underlying etiology. In the United States the typical causes are post-surgical (such as after hemorrhoidectomy, fissurectomy, or fistulec-tomy), neurogenic causes (such as diabetes or multiple sclerosis), Crohn's disease, and the idiopathic variety. The basis for idiopathic fecal incontinence was discussed earlier under descending perineum syndrome. In short, chronic straining and excessive perineal descent is believed to result in pudendal nerve injury and eventual dener-vation of the external sphincter complex. A classification of incon-tinence by cause is given in Table 5.3. Pseudoincontinence (see Table

**Table 5.2** *Instructions for Patients with Pruritus Ani*

1. Our goal is to keep the skin of the anal area clean, dry, and slightly acidic.
2. During bath or shower, wash the outside of the anal area with water. Do not use soap in the anal area (it is alkaline and will increase your discomfort). If a cleansing agent is desired, apply Balneol with fingertips or wet cotton balls. When drying the anal area, avoid abrasive trauma or vigorous rubbing by patting the skin dry with a soft towel or using a hair dryer at low heat.
3. Following each bowel movement, make sure the anal area is clean of any residual stool or moisture. This may be accomplished with a nonalcoholic towelette. Be sure not to leave pads in contact with the skin for prolonged periods. Avoid the use of toilet paper on irritated skin. If afterdrainage persists even after meticulous hygiene, rectal irrigation with a 4-oz syringe bulb and warm water may be useful.
4. In the morning and at bedtime, apply a thin cotton pledget directly in the anal crease. It should be small enough so that you are not conscious of its presence. You may dust the cotton with baby powder or cornstarch if needed. It is important to change the pledget often during the day if it becomes moist.
5. Soaking in a warm sitz bath for 20 minutes can provide relief. Do not add any soaps or skin softeners to the water, and be sure to dry the anal area thoroughly afterward.

5.3) refers to discharge of mucous feces or exudate onto the perineum without incontinence of rectal contents.

During examination, the anus and perineum are inspected for soiling, deformity, scarring, prolapsing hemorrhoids, and rectal prolapse. Surgical incisions, or tears from childbirth, may be seen to divide the true external sphincter. A channel-like defect is seen posteriorly in some patients, creating the "keyhole" deformity. Touching the perianal skin with a sharp pin will elicit a reflex squeeze of the true external sphincter, the "anal wink reflex." Absence of the

*Table 5.2, continued*

6. Maintain a soft, large, and nonirritating stool so that it can pass through the anal canal without causing mechanical or chemical trauma. This may be accomplished by the following:

   a. A bulking agent such as Konsyl, Metamucil, or Citrucil _____ tablespoons in _____ glasses of water of juice _____ times a day.

   b. Eating a high fiber diet that includes 8 to 10 glasses of water or juice a day, plenty of fruits and vegetables, and bran cereal every day.

   c. Avoiding foods that cause bowel irritation, produce mucus, or aggravate drainage; these include dark colas, spicy foods, citrus foods and juices, coffee (regular or decaffeinated), beer, nuts, popcorn, milk, and foods known to produce gas or indigestion. 7-Up, ginger ale, and other light-colored soft drinks may be tolerated.

7. Wearing cotton gloves to bed can be of benefit if you scratch yourself while sleeping.

8. Recurrences are common and to be expected.

9. Don't become despondent over this, just be sure to reconsult your doctor so that appropriate corrections in therapy can be made.

10. You may apply a hydrocortisone cream, but only if it is directed by your physician for use after a cleansing and drying routine.

Reprinted by permission from Beck, Wexner. Fundamentals of anorectal surgery. New York: McGraw-Hill, 1992.

reflex suggests a neurologic deficit. Resting tone and squeeze strength are assessed during digital examination. Palpation is performed for muscular defects and scarring, but the ability of examination to detect disrupted sphincter musculature is limited. The advent of anal ultrasound has significantly altered evolution of fecal incontinence, because it is very safe, rapid, painless, and accurate (Fig. 5.12) in determining the presence of sphincter damage.

**Table 5.3** *Classification of Etiology of Fecal Incontinence*

Incontinence with abnormal sphincter function
> Sphincter injury
>> Obstetric
>>
>> Surgical
>>
>> Traumatic
>>
>> Rectal prolapse
>>
>> Neoplastic
>
> Sphincter denervation
>> Pudendal nerve injury (e.g., forceps delivery)
>>
>> Descending perineum syndrome
>>
>> Chronic constipation
>>
>> Neoplastic infiltration
>>
>> Spinal cord injury
>
> Systemic illness
>> Multiple sclerosis
>>
>> Diabetes
>>
>> Scleroderma

The type of feces that the patient soils is a critical determinant of management. Patients who are incontinent of solid stool nearly always have major sphincter defects, and some will require surgical repair. However, biofeedback should be considered before surgical repair. Patients who are incontinent of liquid stool, but continent of solids, often can be easily managed by manipulation of their stool character.

### Constipation

A variety of different disturbances may cause patients to report constipation. The easiest of these to quantitate is the frequency of bowel movements. Normal individuals pass three or fewer bowel movements per day and three or fewer per week. Patients with extremely infrequent bowel movements ($\leq 1$ bowel movement per week) often have colonic inertia. This can be documented by a colonic transit

*Table 5.3, continued*

---

    Incontinence with normal sphincter function

      Overwhelming diarrhea

      Dementia

      Decreased rectal compliance

        Ulcerative colitis; Crohn's disease

        Radiation proctitis

        Irritable bowel syndrome

    Overflow incontinence

      Impaction

      Encopresis

      Rectal cancer

    Pseudoincontinence

      Mucosal prolapse

      Hemorrhoidal prolapse

      Poor cleansing

      Perineal infections

      Anal cancer

      Fistula

      Incomplete rectal emptying

---

study, in which the patient swallows radiopaque markers followed by plain abdominal x-rays.

Other patients sense the presence of stool in the rectal vault but are unable to expel it. These people have an outlet obstruction type of constipation. They may report using digital disimpaction of stool or vaginal and/or perineal pressure to assist defecation. Occasionally they report extrusion of the rectum with straining (i.e., rectal prolapse). Others may report painful defecation or a simple need to strain with bowel movements.

Initially examination focuses on the degree of perineal descent with straining. During digital examination the puborectalis is pal-

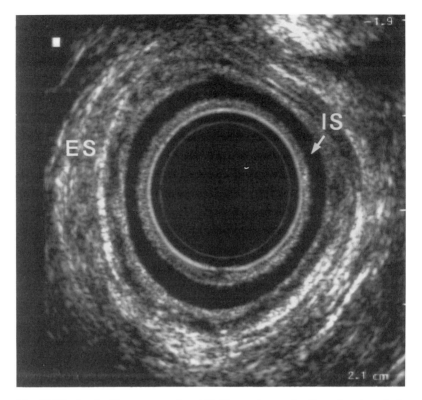

**Fig. 5.12** *Anal ultrasonography. (A) Normal examination showing dark band internal sphincter (IS) and hyperechoic bands of external sphincter (ES).*

pated during straining to make sure that the patient is relaxing the pelvic floor. Failure to relax the pelvic floor during defecations can result in obstructed defecation and has been called "anismus." This is an important diagnosis, as it is common and will respond to biofeedback. However, some normal persons will fail to appropriately relax the pelvic floor during the digital examination because of embarrassment. Therefore, inappropriate contraction of the pelvic floor during a digital examination must be corroborated by demonstrating the finding on another test, such as electromyogram of the anal sphincter or evacuation proctography (defecography) (Fig. 5.13). Treatment of idiopathic constipation is still based initially on

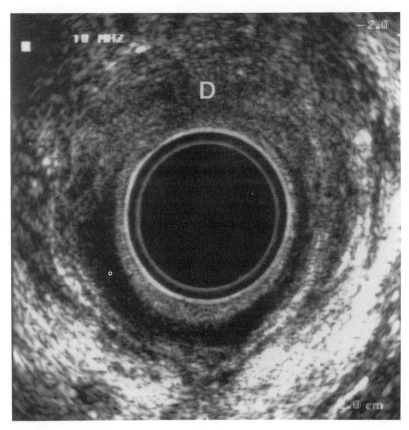

**Fig. 5.12** *Continued. (B) Large anterior defect (D) of both internal and external sphincters.*

fiber supplementation, adequate oral hydration, exercise, and regular bowel habit. Rarely, disabled patients with colonic inertia undergo subtotal colectomy. Certain causes of outlet obstruction constipation warrant therapy, such as very large rectoceles (surgery) and anismus (biofeedback). Palpation of the anterior rectal wall during digital examination will detect a rectocele.

### Chronic Rectal Pain

Chronic rectal pain can in some cases defy diagnosis and resist all forms of therapy. Treatable entities that should be considered in the

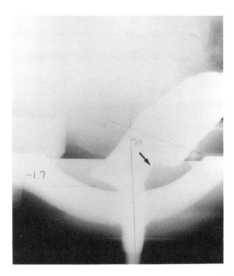

**Fig. 5.13** *Evacuation proctogram during straining to defecate. Anterior is to the left. The anorectal angle is very acute and the puborectalis impression (arrow) is very prominent, resulting in obstructed defecation.*

differential include anal fissure, and anal, rectal, sacral, or pelvic tumors. A difficult syndrome to manage is the levator syndrome. Patients with this syndrome presumably have intermittent development of pelvic floor spasm. No single treatment is consistently effective. Therapy with muscle relaxants, biofeedback, and repeated electrical stimulation of the muscle are each useful in selected patients.

## ◼ PERFORMING THE ANORECTAL EXAMINATION

We will now discuss some of the components of the anorectal examination and describe the presigmoidoscopy examination. With the patient in the left lateral decubitus position, he or she is verbally warned that you are about to begin the examination by visually inspecting the anus and perineum. With one disposable glove on the left hand and two on the right hand, the buttocks are spread and the perineum is visually inspected. Good lighting is essential. The perineal skin is examined for fecal debris, skin excoriation, Monilial or other rashes, fistula orifices, and the presence of skin tags or external hemorrhoids. If the patient has symptoms of a fissure, the index fingers are placed very close to and on either side of the external anal orifice, and the patient is asked to strain. The skin in the distal anal canal is spread by the fingers while the patients' straining everts the squamous mucosa of the anal canal toward the patient. Fissures are typically seen in the posterior (90%) or anterior (10%) anal canal. Prolapsing hemorrhoids or rectal mucosa also may be seen. The index finger of the right hand is well lubricated and the patient is verbally warned that he or she is about to feel some cool jelly in the anal area followed by entrance of your finger. If muscular resistance is felt the patient is asked to strain, which will decrease anal canal pressure and facilitate insertion of the finger. If fibrotic resistance is felt the digital examination should proceed with caution. In males, the prostate gland is palpated for nodules. The rectal mucosa is palpated for masses. The most common mass lesions felt are extremely hypertrophied anal papillae, sometimes called an "anal polyp." These are felt at the proximal end of the anal canal, are pedunculated, and are quite mobile. Any rectal mass will require subsequent verification of its type by direct visual inspection. If the patient has no complaint of constipation or incontinence, there generally will be no need to perform the digital examination during squeezing and straining. If the patient complains of constipation, a careful examination is made for rectocele, and the puborectalis is palpated during straining as a screening examination for proper relaxation of the pelvic floor during straining. If the patient complains of incontinence, then visual and digital inspection must center on distortion of the anal canal and loss of sphincter strength. If the patient complains of prolapse of rectal mucosa or prolapse of the full rectum (Fig. 5.14) and none is elicited in the left lateral decubitus position, then the patient should be examined in the squatting position. After recovery from the sigmoidoscopy, have the patient stand next to the examining table with his or her hands on the table for support. Then have the patient squat and strain to evert the rectum. The examiner must either crouch below the level of the anus to visually inspect for prolapse or examine for prolapse with a mirror. Palpation of the rectum in

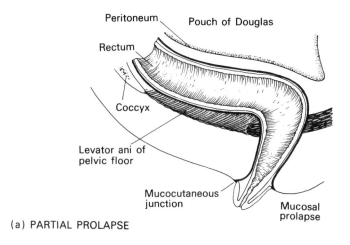

Peritoneum

Pouch of Douglas

Rectum

Coccyx

Levator ani of pelvic floor

Mucocutaneous junction

Mucosal prolapse

(a) PARTIAL PROLAPSE

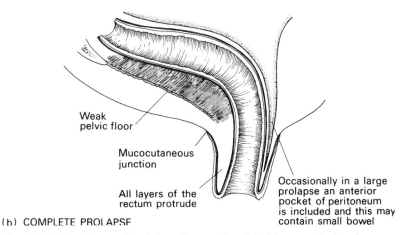

Weak pelvic floor

Mucocutaneous junction

All layers of the rectum protrude

Occasionally in a large prolapse an anterior pocket of peritoneum is included and this may contain small bowel

(b) COMPLETE PROLAPSE

**Fig. 5.14** *Two types of rectal prolapse. (Reprinted by permission from Dunn D, Rawlinson N. Surgical diagnosis and management: a guide to surgical care. 2nd ed. Oxford: Blackwell Science, 1991.)*

the squatting position also may be useful for feeling an enterocele. An enterocele is palpable as a soft mass lesion on the anterior rectal wall with straining.

Following completion of the digital examination, the sigmoidoscope is inserted and the actual sigmoidoscopy is begun. The technique for endoscopic examination of the anus as well as retroflex in the rectum will be covered in the next chapter.

# Bibliography

▼　▼　▼　▼　▼　▼　▼　▼

Church JM. Analysis of the colonoscopic findings in patients with rectal bleeding according to the pattern of their presenting symptoms. Dis Colon Rectum 1991;34:391–395.

> *This is a prospective evaluation of the yield endoscopic evaluation of the lower gastrointestinal tract for different types of bleeding. When blood is mixed with stool, there is a very high probability of cancer. In some patients the history suggests outlet bleeding from an anal source. These individuals have a lower prevalence of colorectal cancer, but a yield is still significant. Thus, evaluation of the colon is necessary.*

Dennison A, Whiston J, Rooney S, et al. A randomized comparison of infrared photocoagulation with bipolar diathermy for the outpatient treatment of hemorrhoids. Dis Colon Rectum 1990;33:32–34.

> *Infrared coagulation is an effective therapy for symptomatic first- and second-degree internal hemorrhoids. The technique is appropriate for office performance by virtually any physician. The advantages of the technique are that the necessary equipment is inexpensive and includes simply an anoscope and the infrared coagulation device, which costs less than $2,000 (Redfield Corp, Montvale, NJ). An alternative is to use bipolar diathermy, which uses an electric current to generate a coagulum of tissue at the end of a cautery-tipped applicator (ACM Bicap, Stamford, CT). The above paper reports a comparison of infrared coagulation to bipolar diathermy; they were found to be equivalent.*

Gooszen HG, Hoedemaker HO, Weterman IT, Keighley MRB. Disordered defaecation. Dordrecht: Martinus Nijhoff, 1987.

> *For those interested in a more detailed understanding of defecation disorders, this little book provides an in-depth introduction. The clinical features of colonic motility, constipation in children and adults, fecal incontinence, and anorectal function testing, including manometry, evacuation proctography, electromyography, and nerve conduction studies, are discussed in detail.*

Goulston KJ, Cook I, Dent OF, and General Practitioners and Specialists Associated with the Concord Hospital Gastroenterology Unit. How important is rectal bleeding in the diagnosis of bowel cancer and polyps? Lancet 1986; 2:261–266.

> *This is another prospective evaluation which showed that neither family physicians nor gastroenterologists in Australia could reliably distinguish the source of rectal bleeding as colonic versus anal by history alone.*

Smith LE. Practical guide to anorectal testing. New York: Igaku-Shoin, 1990.

> *This book takes a different approach to anorectal disease, providing what is essentially a "cookbook" of details on how to perform anorectal function tests. Areas covered include colonic transit studies, several techniques for anorectal manometry, evacuation proctography, electromyography, pudendal nerve, terminal motor latencies, anal sensation, and biofeedback for both constipation and fecal incontinence.*

Whitehead WE, Schuster MM. Anorectal physiology and pathophysiology. Am J Gastroenterol 1987;82:487–497.

> *This an excellent review of anorectal physiology, anorectal testing, and treatment of defecation disorders, such as outlet obstruction, constipation, and fecal incontinence.*

# Technique

▼ ▼ ▼ ▼ ▼ ▼ ▼ ▼

## 6

**T**HIS CHAPTER describes the technique of flexible sigmoidoscopy. After reviewing didactic materials and if possible, a video tape of flexible sigmoidoscopy, the novice should perform a number of examinations under the supervision of a trained endoscopist. The number of supervised examinations needed to achieve competence and independence varies between individuals. In the only rigorous study of this matter, 25 to 30 examinations were needed. However, if beginners had previous experience with rigid sigmoidoscopy, they learned flexible sigmoidoscopy faster and could achieve competence in an average of 15 supervised examinations.

## ■ NORMAL ENDOSCOPIC ANATOMY

The rectum measures 12 to 15 cm in length and extends from the dentate line to the rectosigmoid junction. The rectum is fixed to the sacral wall, and thus the endoscope tip courses posteriorly as it is advanced through the rectum. The lower half of the rectum is the rectal ampulla (Fig. 6.1) and is relatively distensible. The mucosal lining here is smooth, and broad areas of light reflection, termed "highlights," can be seen as the endoscope's tip is moved. The mucosa may appear velvety due to a preponderance of lymphoid tissue. Blood vessels can be readily seen coursing through the ampulla and increase in size with proximity to the anus. At the rectosigmoid junction, blood vessels become less prominent, but remain visible throughout the entire colon. The typical vascular pattern is one of interlacing vascular channels with multiple branches and cross-connections. Inability to identify the vascular pattern indicates a pathologic process. Mucosal edema may cause minute sur-

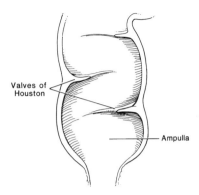

Valves of
Houston

Ampulla

**Fig. 6.1** *Structure of the rectum.*

face irregularities, resulting in fragmentation of the reflected light. The resultant pattern of multiple small reflections is termed "granularity" (Color Plate 1).

Proximal to the rectum, the longitudinal muscle layer of the colon is grouped into three distinct bands, the teniae coli. These tend to give sections of the colon, particularly the transverse colon, a triangular appearance when viewed at endoscopy (Fig. 6.2). In the rectum, however, the longitudinal muscle layer becomes circumferential, making the ampulla round in shape. The proximal half of the rectum contains multiple rectal valves (valves of Houston). These valves are semilunar in shape and typically three in number (see Fig. 6.1). The upper and lower valves usually are located on the left

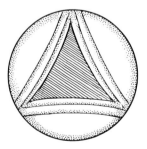

**Fig. 6.2** *The triangular appearance produced by the teniae coli; it is especially prominent in the transverse colon.*

rectal wall and the middle valve is generally on the right wall. This middle valve is located at the level of the peritoneal reflection, usually 11 cm from the external anal verge. The middle valve marks the boundary of lymphatic drainage, as lymphatic drainage above the middle rectal valve courses to the pelvis while below this valve lymph drains to the inguinal nodes. The third or proximal-most valve marks the rectosigmoid junction and typically is 14 to 15 cm from the external anal verge. Once above the fixed anatomy of the rectum the endoscopist cannot identify right, left, anterior, or posterior walls and cannot identify mesenteric from antimesenteric borders.

The sigmoid colon begins at the rectosigmoid junction (Fig. 6.3). It is typically 30 to 40 cm in length, but is sometimes much longer. The sigmoid is notorious for tortuosity and may course through the right abdomen. Endoscopically the lumen is marked by sharp infoldings and angulations.

Relative to the sigmoid, the descending colon (see Fig. 6.3) is

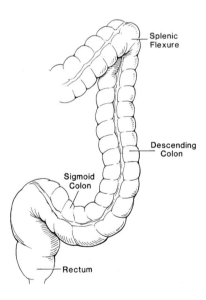

**Fig. 6.3** *The left colon.*

generally straight and tubular. Usually beginning at the pelvic brim, the descending colon extends 25 cm to the splenic flexure. Other than the rectum, the splenic flexure is the most fixed structure in the colon. The descending colon moves anterior and cephalad and the transverse colon moves caudad as they meet at the splenic flexure. This acute angulation, after passing the straight tube of the descending colon, suggests that the splenic flexure has been reached. A round, blue indentation of the spleen also may be seen. Passing the splenic flexure can be confirmed by identifying the characteristic triangular appearance of the transverse colon. Only 15% of 60-cm flexible sigmoidoscopic examinations reach the splenic flexure.

## GOALS OF THE EXAMINATION

The goals of the examination do not include inserting the full 60 cm of instrument in every patient. Many examinations will be performed as screening examinations for colorectal neoplasia. It is important that the patient have a pleasant and not overly painful experience, so that they will speak well of the screening examination to others and so that they will be more likely to return for follow-up examinations themselves. Therefore, the flexible sigmoidoscope should be passed as far as the patient can tolerate with no more than mild discomfort. Beyond this, the goals are safety combined with a careful examination for pathology.

## POSITIONING

After the procedure has been explained to the patient and you are certain that informed consent has been obtained, the patient assumes the left lateral decubitus position. The right leg should be drawn toward the chest, as if the patient were sitting in a chair. The left leg may either remain straight or also can be drawn to the chest (Fig. 6.4). The patient's buttocks should be approximately 2 to 4 inches from the edge of the table. The table height should be adjusted so that the examiner is comfortable. Usually this will involve placing the table at about belt height. It is very uncomfortable and tiring to have to crouch to reach the patient.

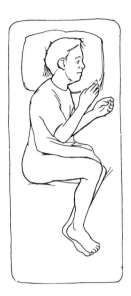

**Fig. 6.4** *Positioning the patient for flexible sigmoidoscopy.*

## ▧ ANAL EXAMINATION AND DIGITAL RECTAL EXAMINATION

Anal and digital rectal examinations should be performed in every patient. Details of the examination were described in Chapter 5.

## ▧ INSERTING THE FLEXIBLE SIGMOIDOSCOPE

The control section of the instrument is placed in the left hand and the tip of the sigmoidoscope is inserted using the right hand. Lubrication is placed along the distal bending portion of the scope, but not over the end of the scope. If the anus is relaxed, the instrument may be inserted straight on (Fig. 6.5). In most cases, however, rather than directly inserting the scope along the axis of the anus, the scope tip is kept at 45° to the axis of the anus (see Fig. 6.5). This creates a smooth rather than blunt entry point for the scope and facilitates entry into the distal anus. After the scope has entered the distal anus, the angle of the scope tip is adjusted to follow the axis of the anal canal. The examiner will have a feeling for the direction of the anal canal from the digital examination. However, it is helpful to

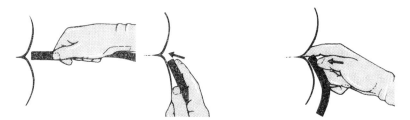

**Fig. 6.5** *Different methods of inserting the sigmoidoscope. (A) The straight-on method may be used if the anus is relaxed. (B) Finger support of the bending section. (C) Tip pushed in as examining finger withdraws. (Reprinted by permission from Cotton PB, Williams CB. Practical gastrointestinal endoscopy. 3rd ed. Oxford: Blackwell Science, 1990.)*

remember that the axis of the anal canal is generally pointed toward the umbilicus (Fig. 6.6). Mild resistance often will be felt in passing the scope through the anus until the tip enters the rectum, when resistance will suddenly drop off. If there is difficulty in passing through the anus, the scope is withdrawn, and the digital examination of the anus is repeated. This will once again dilate and lubricate the anus and refresh the examiners' memory about any ridges

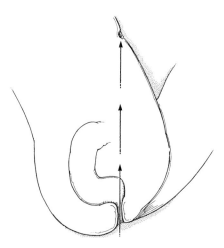

**Fig. 6.6** *The axis of the anus generally points toward the umbilicus.*

or deformities that are palpable in the anal canal. Another attempt at insertion is then performed. Once the examiner feels the scope tip entering the rectum, the outer glove on the right hand is removed and disposed, and the examination begins.

## ■ CONTROL OF INSERTION TUBE

*Two-Person Versus One-Person Technique*

An occasional experienced examiner and many novices prefer to use a two-person technique for scope insertion and withdrawal. In this method the examiner holds the control head in the left hand and uses the right hand to assist in adjusting the directional controls. An assistant holds the shaft of the instrument, and inserts and withdraws it at the examiners' command (Fig. 6.7). It is preferable for the assistant to be able to also visually follow the examination, either on the video screen or with the teaching attachment for a fiberoptic scope. In the one-person technique the examiner holds the control head in the left hand, and inserts and withdraws the instrument shaft with the right hand (Fig. 6.8). Nearly all experts use the one-person technique, and most novices now use the one-person technique from the onset or change to it after a break-in period with the two-person technique.

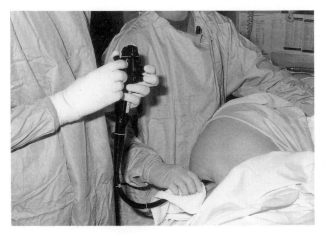

**Fig. 6.7** *The two-person technique of instrument advancement.*

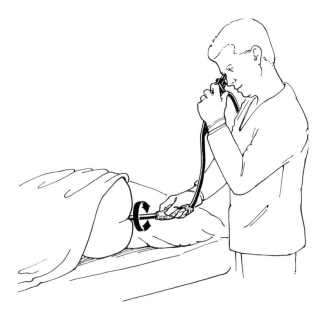

**Fig. 6.8** *"Single-handed" maneuvering of the sigmoidoscope.*

### Directional Controls

The colon is not a straight tube, and it is necessary to turn the sigmoidoscope tip to negotiate colon turns. The examiner's left thumb always controls the up-down directional control. In the two-person technique the examiner can use the right hand to adjust the right-left control. Some examiners who use the one-person technique adjust the right-left directional control with their left thumb (Fig. 6.9). More commonly, however, the right hand is kept on the shaft of the instrument to control insertion and withdrawal, and is taken off the shaft for brief periods to adjust the right-left control as needed.

### Changing Direction

Changing the up-down direction is always controlled by the left thumb and the up-down directional control. Changing the instrument tip direction to the right or left can be achieved by two fundamentally different methods. One is to adjust the right-left control.

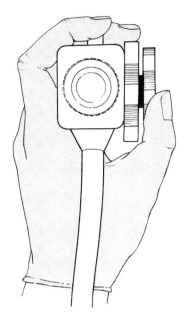

**Fig. 6.9** *The thumb can reach the lateral control knob for right-left deflection if the hand is positioned properly. (Reprinted by permission from Cotton PB, Williams CB. Practical gastrointestinal endoscopy. 3rd ed. Oxford: Blackwell Science, 1990.)*

The other (more advanced) method involves the application of torque to the instrument shaft. Torque rotates the instrument shaft either clockwise or counterclockwise. Torque is applied to the instrument with the right hand by twisting the shaft (Fig. 6.10). Since the shaft often becomes slippery from the lubricant, it should typically be held with either cloth or gauze. A washcloth works well, and should be changed as needed if it becomes soaked with lubricant. Once most of the instrument shaft has been inserted, it becomes difficult to apply torque to the shaft by twisting the shaft with the right hand. Thus, torque is applied by rotating the control head with the left hand and forearm (Fig. 6.11). If a fiberoptic instrument is in use, this may necessitate the examiner bending his or her head to keep the image oriented.

Figure 6.12 shows further how torque can be used to accomplish

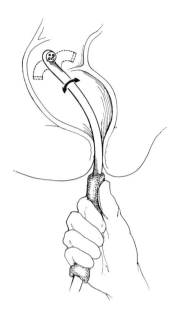

**Fig. 6.10** *Using gauze to grip the instrument shaft, clockwise or counter-clockwise torque is applied (arrow). With the instrument tip deflected in the up or down direction, torque on the instrument shaft will result in right or left turns (dotted lines).*

right-left turns without using the right-left control knobs. This method is sufficiently effective that sigmoidoscopes have been made without right-left controls. However, it is preferable to have right-left controls on the instrument.

### ■ EXAMINING THE RECTUM

The first image obtained is often a "redout." This means that the scope tip is touching the colonic mucosa. An image usually can be obtained most easily by withdrawing the shaft 1 to 2 cm and adjusting the directional controls. The normal rectal mucosa has a salmon color and blood vessels are evident. The instrument is now ready for advancement. Advancing through the rectum is generally easy. The luminal caliber of the rectum is large, and the rectal axis is generally straight. The only obstacles to advancement through the rectum are the rectal valves (valves of Houston). These large folds

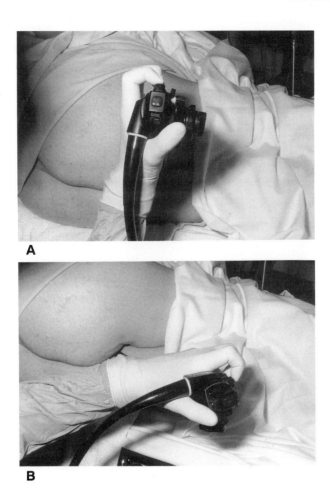

A

B

**Fig. 6.11** *Application of torque by rotation of the control head with the left wrist and forearm. (A) neutral position; (B) torque applied.*

project into the lumen with a crescentic shape. If the scope tip comes up against them, a redout will recur, but the luminal image can be easily obtained again by a short withdrawal of the scope and an adjustment of the directional controls.

## ■ MAINTAINING THE LUMEN

The first obstacle of any difficulty, and often the most problematic point of the examination, is the rectosigmoid junction. Finding the

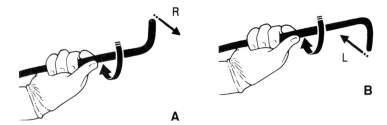

**Fig. 6.12** *With a clockwise shaft twist (A) up-angling moves tip to the right and (B) down-angling moves tip to the left. (Reprinted by permission from Cotton PB, Williams CB. Practical gastrointestinal endoscopy. 3rd ed. Oxford: Blackwell Science, 1990.)*

lumen from this point on requires the examiner to follow several rules for lumen location. Whenever there is difficulty in advancing the scope, the shaft should be withdrawn a few centimeters to examine for one of the following clues.

### Darkness

The lumen will appear dark since it is farther away from the illumination source in the tip of the endoscope. Thus, if tip deflection results in brightening of the visual image, the tip probably is moving closer to the colon wall and the lumen will be in the opposite direction (Fig. 6.13A).

### Fold Shadowing

As the illumination source shines on the haustral folds, the haustral folds cast a shadow. The lumen is behind these folds and in the direction of the shadow (Fig. 6.13B).

### Concentric Ridges

An experienced endoscopist can tell the direction of the lumen by seeing the light reflection from any mucosal fold. This is because the mucosa is stretched over a circular muscle layer. The muscle layer gives the mucosa a curved appearance endoscopically. Although none of the curves forms a full circle, each curve forms an arch which, if extended, would form a circle around the bowel

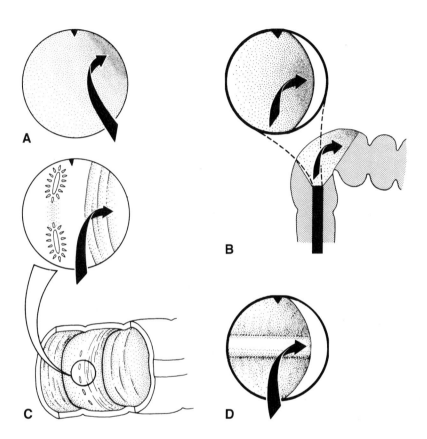

**Fig. 6.13** *(A) Aim at the darkest area. (B) The lumen is in the direction of the shadow cast by the haustral fold. (Reprinted by permission from Cotton PB, Williams CB. Practical gastrointestinal endoscopy. 3rd ed. Oxford: Blackwell Science, 1990.) (C) Aim at the center of the arch formed by the folds, muscle fibers, or reflected "highlights." (Reprinted by permission from Cotton PB, Williams CB. Practical gastrointestinal endoscopy. 3rd ed. Oxford: Blackwell Science, 1990.) (D) At an acute bend follow the longitudinal fold (teniae coli). (Reprinted by permission from Cotton PB, Williams CB. Practical gastrointestinal endoscopy. 3rd ed. Oxford: Blackwell Science, 1990.)*

wall. The direction for tip deflection to the center of that circle is the direction to the center of lumen (Fig. 6.13C).

### Longitudinal Fold

Above the rectum, the longitudinal muscle layer of the colon is grouped into three bundles called the "teniae coli." From the lumen, these bundles may appear to form longitudinal folds, particularly at acute angles. When present, they point out the direction of the lumen (Fig. 6.13D).

### ▦ TIPS FOR INSTRUMENT ADVANCEMENT

A variety of tips are given here for successful advancement of the instrument.

### Unchanging "Redout"

If there is a visual "redout" and tip deflection does not change the redout, then the tip of the scope is stuck against the colon wall. This phenomenon can be reproduced by holding the tip of the scope somewhat firmly against your assistant's hand and moving the tip deflection controls. You will see that the tip of the scope remains firmly against the assistant's hand, while the bending portion and shaft swing in different directions. When this phenomenon is encountered in the colon, the only solution is to withdraw the endoscope and search again for the lumen using the above-mentioned clues.

### Overdistention

You have to use some common sense with air insufflation. You need to put enough air in so that you can distinguish the luminal direction, while at the same time you should try to not continuously insufflate air and overdistend the colon. There are several problems with overdistention. First, although air insufflation is not the most common cause of discomfort, eventually significant air distention of the colon can cause pain. Second, the colon will elongate with air distention and decrease the length of colon that can be effectively intubated. Finally, as the colon becomes distended, the angulations may become more acute and difficult to pass. Suctioning air from a widely distended colon during insufflation can facilitate passage.

## Slide By

In general, it is preferable to keep the lumen in view at all times during insertion. However, at times it is impossible because of a sharp angulation. At that time a slide by maneuver may be needed. The slide by always starts by careful determination of the direction of the luminal turn. The scope is then advanced into the turn and the tip is directed into the turn, followed by gentle advancement. As long as the mucosa is seen to slide by in the direction opposite that of the turn, advancement can continue. Eventually the lumen on the opposite wall of the turn will appear. However, if the mucosa stops sliding by at any time, advancement should be stopped and the instrument should be withdrawn for reassessment of the turn and another attempt. Likewise, if the patient has significant pain, stop, pull back, reassess the direction of the turn, and try again.

## Turn at the Right Time

When you are looking down the lumen and see a turn ahead of you, you must remember that you have not yet reached the turn. A common error made by novices is to begin turning before the scope tip has actually advanced into the turn. The general sequence of passing through the turn is as follows. First, examine the turn and decide what direction the colon is turning. Next, advance the scope tip until the tip is actually in the turn. Adjust the instrument controls and/or the torque in the direction of the turn. Finally, advance the instrument through the turn either under direct vision or via slide by technique.

## Avoid Slip Backs

A constant frustration for the beginner using the one-person technique is slip back of the scope. The frustration begins when the scope tip is advanced into the turn and then the examiner removes the right hand from the instrument shaft to adjust the right-left control and deflect the scope tip in the direction of the turn. Unfortunately, as soon as the right hand leaves the shaft the instrument tip slips back and is no longer in the turn. Now the examiner must re-advance the scope tip into the turn and if he then removes his hand from the shaft again to adjust the right-left control, the scope tip may slip back again. After several tries, frustration may set in. What is needed is a mechanism to keep forward force applied to the shaft while the hand is taken off the shaft to adjust the right-left control. A simple method is to have the assistant hold the shaft and not allow it to slip back. There are two ways to do it without relying on the assistant. The first way depends on having the patient's buttocks placed 2 to 4 inches from the edge of the table. This allows the examiner to lean his or her abdomen forward and press against the shaft of the instrument (Fig. 6.14). This will keep

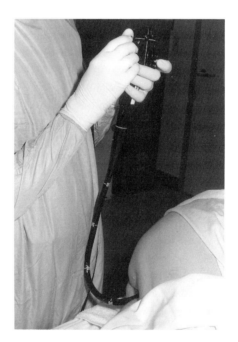

**Fig. 6.14** *When the scope has just started into the sigmoid, the examiner may avoid slip backs by pressing against the shaft with the abdomen.*

enough forward force on the instrument to keep it from slipping back. The second method is more appropriate for slip back occurring deeper in the sigmoid, when more of the shaft has passed the anal canal. In this technique the left hand and arm are used to apply pressure on the control head in the direction of the anus (Fig. 6.15). In summary, to avoid slip back, use the "tummy push" method for the first couple of sigmoid turns when only a small amount of the shaft has passed the anus; later in the examination, use pressure on the control head in the direction of the anus.

### Diverticular Orifices

The examiner must take care not to mistake diverticular orifices for the lumen. Observation often will demonstrate the mucosa in the base of the diverticulum and an absence of haustral folds in the diverticulum (Fig. 6.16). When the tip is against a diverticular orifice it is necessary to withdraw and look for landmarks denoting luminal direction.

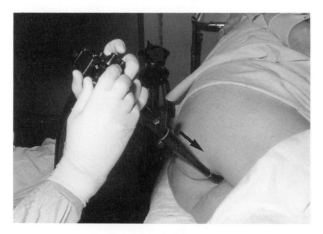

**Fig. 6.15** *When the instrument is nearing full insertion, slip backs are avoided by using the left hand (which is on the control head) and forearm to exert pressure on the control head in the direction of the insertion tube. The arrow shows that the left forearm is directing force on the control head along the axis of the insertion tube (toward the anus).*

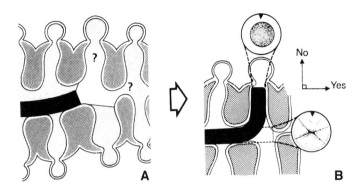

**Fig. 6.16** *(A) The correct path may not be clear in diverticular disease. (Reprinted by permission from Cotton PB, Williams CB. Practical gastrointestinal endoscopy. 3rd ed. Oxford: Blackwell Science, 1990.) (B) A circular view is a diverticulum. Pull back and look at right angles to find the correct direction.*

### *Spasm*

In the sigmoid colon the lumen may collapse or narrow substantially as a result of spasm. The luminal orifice may become a small aperture at the center of converging folds (Fig. 6.17). Either waiting a few moments or gentle steady pressure on the small luminal opening will generally allow passage of the sigmoidoscope.

## ▓ STAYING OUT OF TROUBLE DURING ADVANCEMENT

As we stated earlier, a perforation during a flexible sigmoidoscopy by a primary care physician is particularly likely to lead to a malpractice suit. As experience is gained with flexible sigmoidoscopy, the chances of perforation are extremely low. However, the examiner who is inappropriately aggressive can cause serious problems. Remember that the primary goal of the procedure is not to fully insert the sigmoidoscope. The following rules will help to keep your patients safe and you out of court.

### *Do Not Push Against Fixed Resistance*

This is by far the most important rule to follow. A history of the patient's abdominal surgeries prior to starting will tip you off about

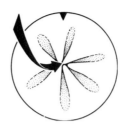

**Fig. 6.17** *Aim at the conversions of folds when spasm is encountered. (Reprinted by permission from Cotton PB, Williams CB. Practical gastrointestinal endoscopy. 3rd ed. Oxford: Blackwell Science, 1990.)*

the possibility of a colon fixed by adhesions. Particularly in women who have had hysterectomies, pelvic adhesions may fix the rectosigmoid colon in position. This fixation will be felt by the hand that is advancing the instrument shaft as unyielding to scope passage.

*Fixed resistance may be encountered even when the lumen is clearly in view* (Fig. 6.18). If you feel that the colon and mesentery are not

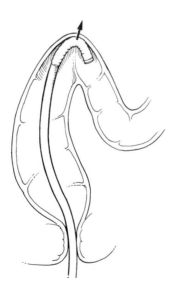

**Fig. 6.18** *Excessive pressure of the bending section on the turn may cause perforation even when the lumen is clearly in view.*

moving in response to your pushing, STOP! There is danger that the pressure point is about to tear the colon open.

### Do Not Advance Blindly

You should never be groping during advancement. The examiner must always either see the lumen or have a clear mental picture of where the lumen is (during a slide by).

### Stop if the Patient Experiences Severe Pain

A pressure sensation or cramping is expected when passing turns. However, if the patient suddenly complains of severe pain it is better to back off, discuss the patient's discomfort with him or her, and reassess whether continued advancement is appropriate.

## ■ SPECIAL MANEUVERS FOR ADVANCEMENT

Performance of special maneuvers for keeping the colonoscope straight and pleating the colon over the scope are very important in colonoscopy. However, they have less importance to flexible sigmoidoscopy. Colonoscopic maneuvers, such as the alpha maneuver (see a colonoscopy text), are seldom necessary or worth the necessary trouble and discomfort to the patient during flexible sigmoidoscopy. A couple of maneuvers can at times be valuable in facilitating scope insertion or increasing the amount of left colon examined during flexible sigmoidoscopy.

### Pullback Maneuver

After passing a turn, the examiner will typically be looking straight down the lumen for a few centimeters. The immediate temptation is to continue advancing the scope. However, passing through the turn often causes a loop to form in the colon (Fig. 6.19A). Therefore, after passing a turn, it is preferable to try to straighten the sigmoidoscope, which in turn will straighten and shorten the colon. The lumen is kept in view during this maneuver by maintaining tip deflection. This is often called "hooking" the turn. Clockwise torque is then applied to the sigmoidoscope and the scope is withdrawn. As the scope is withdrawn the tip of the scope typically will not

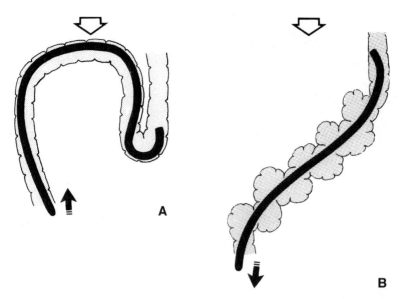

**Fig. 6.19** *(A) During advancement loops may form. Further advancement is facilitated by stopping, "hooking" the turn, and withdrawing the scope with clockwise torque (Reprinted by permission from Cotton PB, Williams CB. Practical gastrointestinal endoscopy. 3rd ed. Oxford: Blackwell Science, 1990.), (B) resulting in shortening and straightening of the colon. (Reprinted by permission from Cotton PB, Williams CB. Practical gastrointestinal endoscopy. 3rd ed. Oxford: Blackwell Science, 1990.)*

move or may actually paradoxically advance forward. As the scope straightens the sigmoid colon will "accordionize" or begin to pleat over the sigmoidoscope (Fig. 6.19B). This results in shortening of the sigmoid colon as the instrument shaft straightens. When the shaft is fully straightened additional withdrawal will start to withdraw the tip. At this point the instrument shaft is typically straight (see Fig. 6.19B) and the instrument can now be re-advanced down the lumen. Repeating this process of hooking just after passing the turn and straightening the instrument with clockwise withdrawal will increase the length of colon that can be examined. In some cases it may be helpful to have the assistant apply firm pressure to the left lower quadrant or left mid-abdomen to prevent formation of a loop during advancement and to thereby keep the scope tip advancing.

For the most part, clockwise torque is the most useful direction during flexible sigmoidoscopy. Counterclockwise torque is seldom beneficial.

### Jiggling

During a slide by, jiggling the instrument in and out with rapid (2 to 5/sec) movement may help the scope tip slide by. If jiggling is used during slide by, the same rules apply regarding stopping the slide by for significant discomfort or failure of the mucosa to slide by. Variations of this in-and-out movement as well as wiggling the tip of the instrument with up-down controls are occasionally helpful in further advancing the scope tip.

### ▓ WITHDRAWAL

Withdrawal is the most important part of the examination; this is the time when careful examination is performed. The importance of being thorough cannot be overemphasized. Although a couple of radiologic reports have documented missing colon cancers with flexible endoscopy, this occurrence is probably becoming less frequent as instruments are progressively improved. With modern instruments, therefore, the sensitivity for detection of cancers and large polyps is extremely high. The miss rate for small polyps is probably approximately 15%. With the scope fully inserted, the typical location of the scope tip is near the sigmoid-descending colon junction. Only 16% of 60-cm flexible sigmoidoscopy examinations will actually reach the splenic flexure. Therefore, the term "left colonoscopy," as applied to 60-cm flexible sigmoidoscopy, is a misnomer.

During withdrawal, the examiner strives to keep the lumen in the center of the visual field. In the one-person technique the right hand is kept on the instrument shaft and the right-left directional control is kept in the free or unlocked position. A combination of torquing the instrument shaft and adjusting the up-down directional control is used to keep the lumen in the center of the field. Forward pressure is applied to the instrument shaft using the right hand whenever the scope tip begins to slip back too suddenly, so that a section of the colon might not be carefully examined. In general, a slight rocking of the instrument shaft by torquing the instrument two or three times per second from right to left while pulling backward on the scope will cause the colon to slip slowly off the tip of the instrument and present itself for examination (Fig. 6.20).

As the scope is withdrawn past a turn, a fold may suddenly present itself in front of the sigmoidoscope and cause a redout. These redouts can be avoided by anticipating the direction from which the fold will appear. For example, if the lumen is in the center of the field while the left thumb has moved the up-down directional control in the up direction, then as the scope is withdrawn the next fold will appear from the up direction (Fig. 6.21). As the fold starts to appear the examiner makes the necessary downward adjustment to keep the lumen in the center of the field and avoid the redout. With experience, the examiner will achieve sufficient control of the speed of tip withdrawal with the right hand and sufficient speed of directional control with the left thumb so that redouts will seldom occur during withdrawal. If a redout does occur during withdrawal around a curve, it is best to re-advance the instrument through the curve.

A frustrating experience for the beginner occurs when an angulation in the colon is so sharp that a redout cannot possibly be

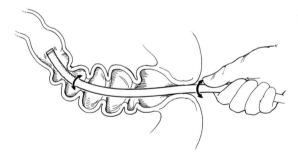

**Fig. 6.20** *Gentle rocking and/or torquing of the instrument during withdrawal encourages the accordionized colon to slip gradually rather than suddenly off the sigmoidoscope tip. This helps prevent the need for reinsertion to examine bowel that slipped by too quickly.*

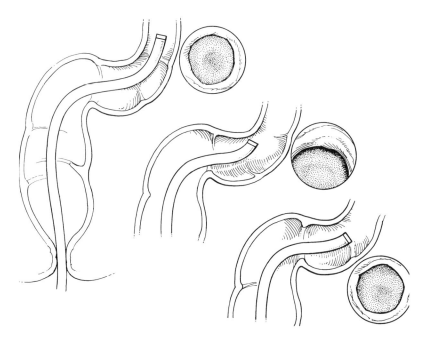

**Fig. 6.21** *In the left panel, the endoscope tip is deflected in the up direction during withdrawal. The examiner can anticipate, therefore, that the next fold will appear in the upper aspect of the visual field (center panel). This anticipation facilitates rapid downward deflection to maintain the lumen in the center of the visual field (right panel).*

avoided during withdrawal. In this case some of the mucosa just proximal to the angulation will not be visualized during withdrawal. Under these circumstances the entire turn often can be well-visualized by reinserting the sigmoidoscope through the turn and examining the turn during insertion. During insertion the bend in the instrument shaft will change the contour of the turn so that the mucosa that was invisible during withdrawal will come into view.

One area where sizable lesions may be missed is behind the rectal valves of Houston. The reason is that the valves often are sufficiently prominent to hide a large area of mucosa on their proximal side (Fig. 6.22). Therefore, as the valves are passed during withdrawal, it is best to reinsert the instrument until its tip has passed

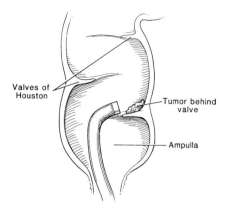

Valves of Houston

Tumor behind valve

Ampulla

**Fig. 6.22** *The careful examiner looks behind haustral folds. It is particularly important to look behind rectal valves.*

the valve and then look behind the valve by either torquing the instrument and using up-down deflection or using the right-left control. Using these careful techniques, the instrument is brought out all the way to the anus. The experienced examiner will feel comfortable that more than 95% of the mucosal surface has been examined and that nothing of significant size has been missed.

### ▓ RETROFLEXION

Retroflexion is a maneuver for turning the scope 180° in the rectum and examining the internal anal verge and the adjacent rectal mucosa. The purpose of retroflexion is that this area can hide significant lesions that may be difficult to see on the forward view. Retroflexion should not be attempted if the luminal diameter of the rectum appears small. A typical situation in which this is encountered is ulcerative colitis. Under these circumstances an attempt at retroflexion often will be unsuccessful and will result in significant pain. In most normal individuals a retroflexion can be performed and is very helpful if an assessment for internal hemorrhoids is needed.

The technique for retroflexion is as follows. After careful inspection on withdrawal all the way to the anus, the sigmoidoscope is then reinserted into the rectum until the 10-cm bending portion is fully past the external anal verge. The directional controls are then flexed in the maximum up and maximum left direction and the right-left control is locked. The right hand is then placed under the instrument shaft with the palm facing up. The instrument is then simultaneously advanced a short distance into the rectum and rotated 180° counterclockwise so that the palm is facing down (Fig. 6.23). If resistance is encountered or the scope cannot be visualized coming through the anus, the examiner should stop, withdraw the instrument, reassess, and try again. Once in the retroflexed position, additional torque in either direction can be helpful to visualize the entire circumference of the internal anal verge and the adjacent rectal mucosa.

## ■ ADDITIONAL TIPS FOR GOOD VISUALIZATION

The flexible sigmoidoscope is designed to optimize your visualization of the colonic mucosa. During withdrawal the examiner can be more liberal with air insufflation. In fact, it is essential to use adequate air insufflation to keep the lumen inflated.

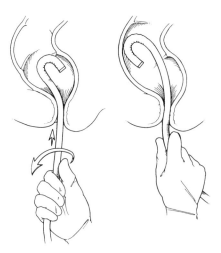

**Fig. 6.23** *Technique for retroflexion. With the tip deflected in the maximum up and left direction, advance and apply counterclockwise torque (left panel), resulting in a retroflexed view of the anus (right panel).*

The image should be kept crystal clear at all times. This is done by liberal use of the water insufflation valve whenever the image becomes cloudy.

Solid material retained in the colon often cannot be removed with suction. Pools of liquid and semisolids often can be removed by suctioning, allowing visualization of the mucosa under the liquid. Keep in mind that the suction port is at the 5 o'clock position in your endoscopic field. Therefore, pools of liquid are most easily suctioned if the instrument is rotated so that the liquid is at the 5 o'clock area of the visual field (Fig. 6.24). This may not be possible or easy to achieve, particularly early in the examiner's experience. If the pool to be suctioned is at the 5 o'clock position, the most efficient suctioning method is to deflect the scope tip so that the 5 o'clock portion of the field is just below the air fluid interface. This allows the examiner to watch as the pool is suctioned from the colon and to stop the suctioning just before mucosa is sucked into the channel.

When mucosa is suctioned into the channel, it can be safely cleared by simple withdrawal of the instrument a few centimeters. This often will leave a suction artifact on the mucosa that will initially appear as a polyp. However, with air insufflation and a few moments of observation this "suction polyp" will quickly disappear.

If the walls of the colon are covered with a thin layer of stool, the material can be cleared by flushing a volume of fluid down the biopsy channel of the sigmoidoscope. In Pentax and Fujinon sigmoidoscopes, a separate "water jet" channel is available to wash

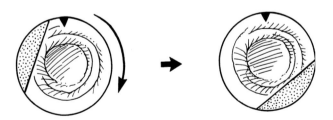

**Fig. 6.24** *(A) If a pool of fluid is in poor position for suctioning, (B) rotation of the instrument shaft will position the pool at 5 o'clock.*

material off the mucosa. Simethicone should be added to the wash fluid to prevent formation of bubbles in the colonic lumen. If such mucosal coating is extensive, however, attempts to clear it through the sigmoidoscope generally are futile. It is best to either withdraw the scope, administer another enema, and then try again, or to reschedule the examination.

At times suctioning will result in a piece of solid material plugging the end of the biopsy channel. This fecal debris generally can be seen at the 5 o'clock location in the visual field. It can be quickly cleared by injection of a small volume of air or water down the biopsy channel.

## ■ TAKING BIOPSY SPECIMENS

Performance of mucosal biopsies with endoscopic forceps generally is a safe procedure (Fig. 6.25). Contraindications include coagulopathy and biopsy of what is potentially a vascular structure, such as a rectal varix or hemorrhoid. It is preferable to use the largest forceps that will pass through the instrument channel. Biopsy specimens can and should be taken from the normal mucosa in patients with chronic diarrhea.

The biopsy forceps will enter the field from the 5 o'clock position. Therefore, it is preferable to keep the 5 o'clock aspect of the

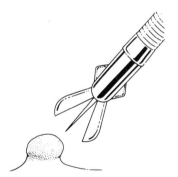

**Fig. 6.25** *A needled biopsy forceps about to grasp a small polyp. (Reprinted by permission from Cotton PB, Williams CB. Practical gastrointestinal endoscopy. 3rd ed. Oxford: Blackwell Science, 1990.)*

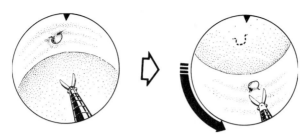

**Fig. 6.26** *(A) If a lesion is difficult to reach with the forceps, (B) a 180° rotation of the straightened shaft makes it easy to reach without losing the view. (Reprinted by permission from Cotton PB, Williams CB. Practical gastrointestinal endoscopy. 3rd ed. Oxford: Blackwell Science, 1990.)*

visual field toward the lumen while the forceps are pushed through. This will help to prevent the forceps from being pushed directly into a diverticulum or ulcer that might perforate. If a polyp is difficult to reach, rotation of the instrument shaft by a combination of torquing and tip deflection can place the polyp in the 5 o'clock position, facilitating the approach to the polyp (Fig. 6.26).

Because the biopsy forceps are passed through the suction channel, suction is diminished while the forceps are in use.

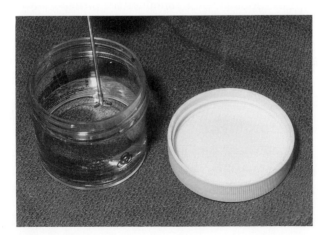

**Fig. 6.27** *Shaking the open forceps in a formalin container will usually dislodge the specimen.*

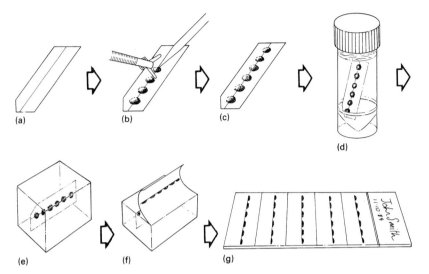

**Fig. 6.28** *Stages in placing biopsy samples on filter paper, orienting, fixing, sectioning, and mounting. (Reprinted by permission from Cotton PB, Williams CB. Practical gastrointestinal endoscopy. 3rd ed. Oxford: Blackwell Science, 1990.)*

Biopsy specimens should be placed in formalin for fixation. Many endoscopists accomplish this by opening the forceps tips containing the specimen in a container for formalin and shaking the forceps until the specimen dislodges from the forceps (Fig. 6.27). However, it is preferable to tweeze the specimens from the open forceps with a needle and orient them onto a piece of filter paper (Fig. 6.28). The filter paper is then placed in formalin for eventual sectioning and mounting (see Fig. 6.28).

## ■ CONCLUSION

You are now armed with the essential technical details of performing flexible sigmoidoscopy. In the next chapter we will review the common pathologic findings.

# Bibliography

▼　▼　▼　▼　▼　▼　▼　▼

Hawes RH, Lehman GA, Hast J, et al. Training resident physicians in fiber-optic sigmoidoscopy: how many supervised examinations are required to achieve competence? Am J Med 1986;80:465–470.

*Resident physicians were judged to be competent in flexible sigmoidoscopy after an average of 25 to 30 supervised examinations. If they had previous experience with rigid sigmoidoscopy they learned faster and were judged to be competent after 15 supervised flexible examinations.*

Hixson L, Fennerty MB, Sampliner R, et al. Prospective blinded trial of the colonoscopic miss rate of large colorectal polyps. Gastrointest Endosc 1991;37:125–127.

*Even modern colonoscopists miss approximately 15% of small polyps. It is clearly better to be slow and careful during withdrawal, but even then the examination cannot be expected to be perfect.*

Laufer I, Smith NCW, Mullens JE. The radiologic demonstration of colorectal polyps undetected by endoscopy. Gastroenterology 1976;70:167–170.

*The second most common reason to be sued for the performance of flexible sigmoidoscopy is to miss a diagnosis. If this ever happens, you will want to be aware of this report, as well as the report of Miller and Lehman. Although they are old references, they document that experienced examiners have missed cancer.*

Lehman GA, Buchner DM, Lappas JC. Anatomical extent of fiberoptic sigmoidoscopy. Gastroenterology 1983;84:806–808.

*A group of patients undergoing 60-cm flexible sigmoidoscopy had metal clips placed on the wall of the colon and then underwent barium enema examination. This study showed that the average extent of 60-cm flexible sigmoidoscopy was the sigmoid descending colon junction, and only 16% of examinations reached the splenic flexure.*

Miller RE, Lehman G. Polypoid colonic lesions undetected by endoscopy. Radiology 1978;129:295–297.

# Findings at Flexible Sigmoidoscopy

▼　▼　▼　▼　▼　▼　▼　▼

## 7

**A** N IMPORTANT differentiation for the examiner to be able to make is normal versus abnormal. The normal colonic mucosa is salmon colored and blood vessels in the submucosa are readily evident. These vessels arborize into very tiny vessels. These vessels are in general considerably more prominent in the rectum than in the sigmoid colon. The luminal diameter of the sigmoid is less than that of the rectum.

## ▉ POLYPS AND CANCER

Neoplasia is the most important finding at flexible sigmoidoscopy. In general, the chance of finding cancer is related heavily to the indication for the procedure. Therefore, sigmoidoscopy will detect a cancer in 5% to 10% of patients who present with rectal bleeding, but in only one in 500 screening examinations. Cancers generally are easily distinguished by their size, their irregular and/or ulcerated surface, and their color, which often is red or even a purple hue. Polypoid cancers (Color Plate 7) (Fig. 7.1) may, however, be small lesions. This emphasizes the importance of examining behind haustral folds and particularly behind rectal valves. Annular or "apple-core" lesions (Color Plate 8) (Fig. 7.2) are considered cancer until proven otherwise. Edema or angulation at the distal edge of a cancer occasionally will make visualization and biopsy of tumor tissue impossible. Referral of such strictures for additional evaluation is appropriate.

The chance of finding colonic polyps is more dependent on demographic factors, such age and gender, than the indication for

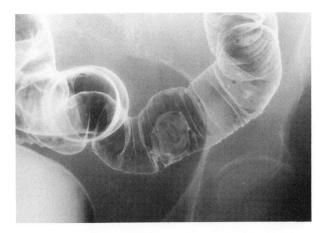

**Fig. 7.1** *Double-contrast barium enema examination showing polypoid cancer. (Courtesy Dr John Lappas.)*

the procedure. Thus, although large colonic polyps can cause rectal bleeding, most colon polyps are asymptomatic. Patients in their sixth decade of life are about twice as likely to have adenomatous polyps as patients 10 years younger. However, after the seventh decade the prevalence of adenomas no longer increases with age. In

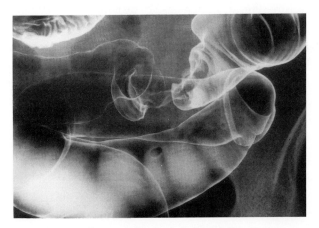

**Fig. 7.2** *Double-contrast barium enema examination demonstrating annular sigmoid carcinoma. (Courtesy Dr John Lappas.)*

addition, males are more likely than females to have adenomas. An asymptomatic 70-year-old man is approximately four to five times as likely as a 50-year-woman to have an adenomatous polyp.

Histologic types of colon polyps are listed below:

Neoplastic
 Adenoma
 Carcinoma
Nonneoplastic
 Hyperplastic
 Juvenile (retention)
 Inflammatory (pseudopolyp)

For practical purposes, the two types of colonic polyps with which examiners should be most familiar are adenomas and hyperplastic polyps. The larger a polyp is, the more likely it is an adenomatous rather than hyperplastic polyp.

Adenomas are neoplastic lesions and can give rise to colorectal cancer. More than 95% of colorectal cancers are believed to arise from adenomatous polyps. The larger an adenomatous polyp becomes, the greater the probability that it already contains at least a focus of cancer. Histologically, adenomas may be classified as tubular or villous. Tubular adenomas have an organized glandular architecture (Fig. 7.3) They tend to be smaller than villous adenomas and are less likely to have severe dysplasia or invasive cancer. Villous adenomas exhibit a frond-like glandular architecture (see Fig. 7.3). If the overall structure of an adenoma is greater than 75% tubular, the pathologist will designate it a tubular adenoma. If an adenoma has more than 75% villous elements, it will be designated a villous adenoma. If the adenoma is a mixture of tubular and villous elements it is designated as a tubulovillous (or sometimes villoglandular) adenoma. The risk of severe dysplasia or invasive carcinoma in tubulovillous adenomas is intermediate between that of tubular and villous adenomas. Endoscopically, adenomas also are classified as pedunculated (having a stalk) or sessile (Figs. 7.4 and 7.5). Sessile adenomas are more likely to be malignant and to have invasion than pedunculated adenomas of comparable size. From the viewpoint of

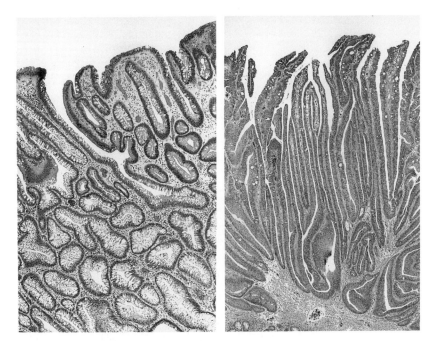

**Fig. 7.3** *(A) Photomicrograph of tubular adenoma. There are irregular, branching glands lined by atypical (dysplastic) columnar cells. (Courtesy Dr O.W. Cummings.) (B) Photomicrograph of a villous adenoma. Villi or fronds are present on over 75% of the surface. There is a higher degree of dysplasia. (Courtesy Dr O.W. Cummings.)*

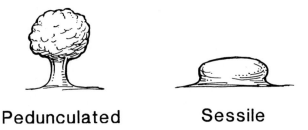

Pedunculated                    Sessile

**Fig. 7.4** *Polyps may be endoscopically classified as pedunculated (left) or sessile (right).*

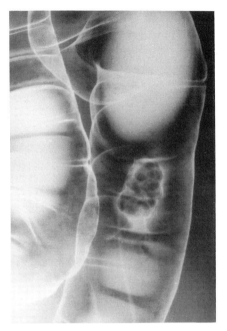

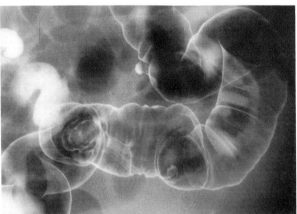

**Fig. 7.5** *Double-contrast barium enema examinations demonstrating pedunculated adenomas with short (A) and long (B) stalks. (Courtesy Dr John Lappas.)*

the sigmoidoscopist, however, this distinction has little importance, as either type of adenoma should be resected. Table 7.1 lists the relationship of polyp size to the probability that a polyp is an adenoma rather than a hyperplastic polyp, and secondly that it is an adenoma that contains cancer.

Hyperplastic polyps are small, generally sessile, and tend to be pale in color (Color Plate 9), but can be red (Color Plate 10). Typically they are less than 5 mm in size, although considerably larger hyperplastic polyps are occasionally encountered. In general, hyperplastic polyps are distributed more toward the very distal colon than are adenomas. Because of their distal distribution, the sigmoidoscopist encounters and must deal with hyperplastic polyps on a regular basis. Hyperplastic polyps are not neoplasms (Fig. 7.6). They do not transform into either adenomas or cancer. Although adenomas (Color Plates 11 through 17) are more likely than hyperplastic polyps to be red in color, it is impossible to reliably distinguish small adenomas from hyperplastic polyps based on their appearance alone. Although adenomas and hyperplastic polyps tend to cluster spatially, the current belief is that hyperplastic polyps are not strong markers for adenomatous polyps in the proximal colon. Therefore, in asymptomatic patients, detection of a hyperplastic polyp is not currently considered an indication for colonoscopy. Generally, accurate distinction of a hyperplastic from adenomatous polyp requires

**Table 7.1** *Relationship of Polyp Size to the Probability That a Polyp Is an Adenoma Versus Hyperplastic and That the Polyp Contains Cancer*

| Size (mm) | Adenoma (%) | Cancer (%) |
|---|---|---|
| 2–3 | <50 | Rare |
| 4–5 | 50 | Rare |
| 6–9 | 85 | 1 |
| 10–20 | >95 | 5 |
| >20 | >95 | >30 |

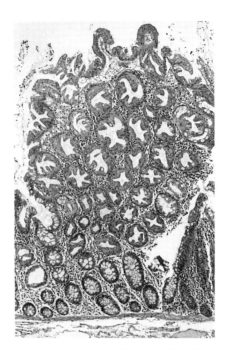

**Fig. 7.6** *Photomicrograph of a hyperplastic polyp. Note the sawtooth surface. The glands have round to oval outlines but serrated lumenal surfaces. The glands are lined by nondysplastic epithelium. (Courtesy Dr O.W. Cummings.)*

taking a biopsy specimen of the polyp. However, disappearance of small polyps with air insufflation is a reliable predictor that the polyp is hyperplastic. Such disappearing polyps can be safely ignored.

What should be done when colon polyps are detected by flexible sigmoidoscopy? One approach is to refer all patients with polyps detected at flexible sigmoidoscopy for colonoscopy. However, this will result in colonoscopy of a significant number of patients who only have distal hyperplastic polyps at flexible sigmoidoscopy. There is insufficient data to support these lesions being important markers for large adenomas or cancers in the proximal colon. A more cost-effective approach is to take biopsy samples from polyps that are ≤ 5 mm in size. A significant number of these small polyps are hyperplastic polyps. If the pathology report returns showing only hyperplastic polyps, then the patient need not be referred for colonoscopy. If an adenoma is detected by the pathologic evaluation, the patient should be referred for colonoscopy.

If a polyp detected at flexible sigmoidoscopy is larger than 5 mm in size, then it is probably more cost-effective to simply refer the patient for colonoscopy. The rationale for this is that the great majority of polyps larger than 5 mm in size are adenomas. If such polyps are biopsied, then the patient incurs a pathologic examination fee for biopsy of the polyp during flexible sigmoidoscopy, and in most cases will incur a second fee for pathologic examination of the same polyp when the polyp is removed during colonoscopy. An algorithm depicting this approach is shown in Figure 7.7. Once again, small polyps that disappear with air insufflation can be assumed to be hyperplastic and no biopsy is needed.

Obviously the algorithm presented in Figure 7.7 is dependent on the ability of the examiner to measure the size of the polyp. Unfortunately, there is no reliable method for accomplishing this task. Most gastroenterologists believe that primary care physicians overestimate the size of polyps during flexible sigmoidoscopy. However, when the subject is rigorously studied, it is found that both primary care physicians and gastroenterologists generally underestimate the size of polyps. Probably the most reliable method cur-

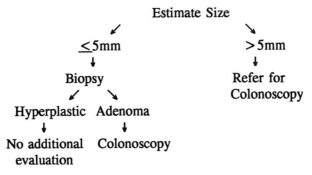

**Fig. 7.7** *Management of polyps detected at screening flexible sigmoidoscopy.*

rently available to estimate the size of a polyp is to take an open biopsy forceps of known width and actually push the forceps up against the polyp to compare polyp size to the known size of the open forceps (see Fig. 7.7). Our own experience is that for polyps in the 2- to 7-mm range, one can learn from this technique to visually estimate the size of polyps with an accuracy of 1 to 2 mm.

## ■ DIVERTICULOSIS

The prevalence of diverticulosis (Fig. 7.8) increases with age in most Western countries. The pathogenesis of diverticulosis is a diet that is low in fiber. People who ingest diets rich in fiber do not develop diverticular disease. Inadequate dietary fiber leads to small scybalous stools. The colon develops high intraluminal pressures because of these small stools and the consequent low intraluminal volume. (Remember Laplace's law?) In response to these high pressures, the muscle layer in the wall of the colon eventually becomes hypertro-

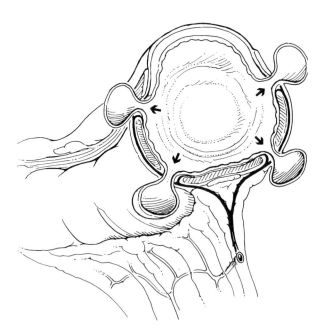

**Fig. 7.8** *Diverticulosis of the colon.*

phied. With progressive hypertrophy, haustral folds on opposite walls of the sigmoid may touch, resulting in segmentation. Segmentation is believed to further increase the tendency for high intraluminal pressure. The high intraluminal pressures eventually cause herniation of the mucosa through the muscle layer of the colon (Fig. 7.9). The point at which the herniation occurs is the point at which small arteries penetrate the muscular layer from the serosal surface to enter the submucosa (Fig. 7.10). At these points there is a natural weakness in the wall. Diverticulosis is most prominent in the sigmoid colon, which has the smallest intraluminal volume of any colonic segment, and is rare in the rectum. Diverticulosis often is seen best during insertion of the sigmoidoscope (Color Plate 18) rather than withdrawal. During withdrawal the sigmoid colon often is straightened over the sigmoidoscope, and the orifices of diverticula tend to lie more tangential to the field of vision.

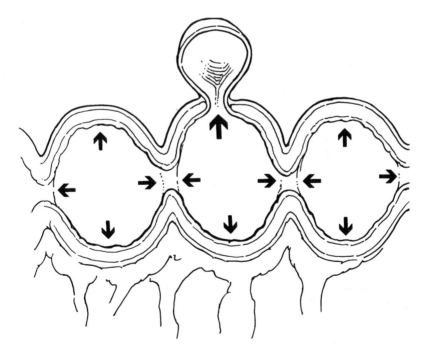

**Fig. 7.9** *The pathogenesis of diverticulosis involves high intraluminal pressures that develop in response to inadequate dietary fiber.*

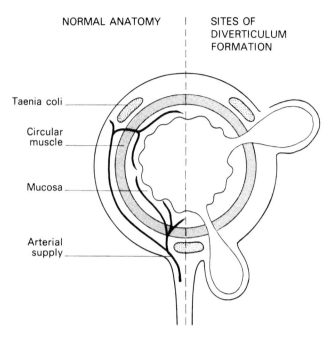

NORMAL ANATOMY | SITES OF DIVERTICULUM FORMATION

Taenia coli

Circular muscle

Mucosa

Arterial supply

**Fig. 7.10** *Diverticula form on the antimesenteric colonic borders at points of natural weakness in the muscle wall where arteries penetrate from the serosa to the submucosa. (Reprinted by permission from Dunn DC, Rawlinson N. Surgical diagnosis and management: a guide to surgical care. 2nd ed. Oxford: Blackwell Science, 1991.)*

Most diverticulosis is asymptomatic. Clinical syndromes associated with diverticulosis are as follows:

- Asymptomatic diverticulosis
- Painful diverticular disease
- Diverticular bleeding
- Diverticulitis

If detected during a screening examination, patients should be informed that they have diverticulosis. This may be helpful to them if they ever develop symptoms of diverticulitis or massive colonic bleeding. The patient should be instructed to increase his or her dietary fiber to retard the development of new diverticula. Patients with asymptomatic diverticulosis are sometimes instructed to avoid foods containing small seeds or other indigestible particles. The rationale is that these particles could become lodged in a diverticulum and result in diverticulitis. There is no real clinical data to support this hypothesis, and we do not bring it up with patients. If patients ask about it, we explain the theory behind the recommendation and note to the patient that the theory is unproven. The decision can then be left to the patient.

Diverticulosis can be an explanation for abdominal pain in the absence of signs of infection. This syndrome is called "painful diverticular disease" and presents as left lower quadrant pain with altered bowel habit and a sometimes tender sigmoid colon on abdominal palpation. However, there is no fever or elevation of the white blood cell count. This syndrome is a variant of irritable bowel syndrome. In older patients with new-onset abdominal pain in whom a flexible sigmoidoscopy shows only diverticulosis, it is preferable to follow up with an air contrast barium enema or refer the patient for colonoscopy to rule out colon cancer at a site more proximal to the extent of flexible sigmoidoscopy.

Diverticulitis is a syndrome of lower abdominal pain, fever, and elevated white blood count resulting from infection of a diverticulum. A microperforation develops in the base of the diverticulum, but is contained by an inflammatory response that "walls off" the diverticulum. In general, flexible sigmoidoscopy is relatively contraindicated in patients with acute diverticulitis. Air insufflation during sigmoidoscopy could theoretically rupture the contained perforation, resulting in free perforation and peritonitis. In reality this risk is probably very low. However, the diagnosis should be made on clinical grounds and the patient treated with antibiotics. An abdominal computed tomography scan (Fig. 7.11) often is the most useful initial diagnostic test, since it can confirm the inflammatory process in the sigmoid colon as well as visualize any abscess that might require percutaneous or surgical drainage. If the diagnosis is in doubt, a barium enema can be used, which may demonstrate a fistula tract leading from the base of the diverticulum (Fig. 7.12).

Patients presenting with massive hematochezia are most often bleeding from diverticulosis. The pathogenesis of diverticular bleed-

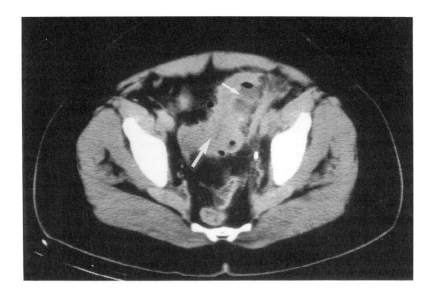

**Fig. 7.11** *An abdominal computed tomography scan demonstrates sigmoid thickening (small arrow), a mass in the mesentery, and a diverticular abscess (large arrow). (Courtesy Dr John Lappas.)*

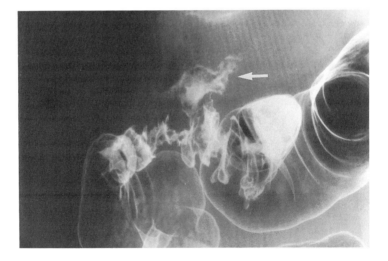

**Fig. 7.12** *Double-contrast barium enema examination demonstrating diverticulitis. There is spasm and narrowing. The diagnostic feature is the fistula tract (arrow) heading from the base of the infected diverticulum. (Courtesy Dr John Lappas.)*

ing in these patients is the stretching of a submucosal artery in the base of the diverticulum. Flexible sigmoidoscopy generally is the first diagnostic test performed, but should most often be performed by an expert. The presence of active hemorrhage in the colon can make the examination very challenging.

## COLITIS

The endoscopic appearance of acute infectious colitis from *Shigella* sp, *Campylobacter* sp, or *Salmonella* sp amebiasis can be difficult or impossible to distinguish from chronic idiopathic ulcerative colitis. As discussed earlier, biopsy samples can usually differentiate acute self-limiting colitis from idiopathic inflammatory bowel disease. When flexible sigmoidoscopy is used to assess the severity of ulcerative colitis, the findings are of secondary importance to the patients' clinical condition. Ulcerative colitis can be judged as quiescent, mild, moderate, or severe by either clinical (Table 7.2) or endoscopic grounds. However, the correlation between the two is less than perfect. Thus, some patients with clinically very significant symptoms will have very mild changes endoscopically. On the other hand, approximately 10% of patients with severe endoscopic ulcerative colitis are asymptomatic. In most patients a combination of clinical findings and endoscopic findings are considered in decision making.

Quiescent endoscopic disease means no endoscopic evidence of active inflammation. However, there may be absence or distortion of the normal vascular pattern and a pale, thin appearance to the mucosa, often referred to as "atrophy."

Mild endoscopic disease (Color Plate 1) is characterized by granularity, erythema, and mild friability. Granularity is recognized endoscopically as a mucosal pattern of many tiny white dots. The dots are reflected light from the illumination source in the endoscope. This pattern of reflected light is caused by a fine nodularity of the mucosal surface, which is itself the result of mucosal edema. Friability refers to the tendency of mucosa to bleed when it is touched by the scope.

Moderate ulcerative colitis involves mucopus in the lumen and

**Table 7.2** *Clinical Classification of the Severity of Ulcerative Colitis*

Mild disease
> Ambulatory patient
> ≤5 stools per day; small amounts of blood
> Mild abdominal cramping
> Afebrile
> Normal hemoglobin, albumin

Moderate disease
> 5–10 stools per day; regular bleeding
> Considerable cramping
> Intermittent low-grade fever
> Mild anemia; hypoalbuminemia

Severe disease
> >10 stools; often passes only blood
> Dehydration present
> Frequently febrile
> Marked anemia; hypoalbuminemia

ulcerations ≤ 5 mm in size, in addition to all features of mild disease. The very presence of mucopus in the lumen is equivalent to ulceration. In other words, mucopus implies that at least pinpoint ulcerations are present, even if they are not endoscopically visible.

Severe disease (Color Plate 2) has the features of moderate disease, although ulcerations are greater than 5 mm in size and the mucosa is bleeding spontaneously so that blood is seen in the lumen when the rectum is first entered. The management of ulcerative colitis is beyond the scope of this book.

## ▓ CROHN'S COLITIS

Crohn's disease of the colon may spare the rectum and in approximately half of patients the entire flexible sigmoidoscopy will be negative. The earliest lesion of Crohn's disease is the aphthous ulcer.

Aphthous ulcers are 1 to 2 mm in diameter and are surrounded by erythema. The mucosa between the aphthous ulcers may appear perfectly normal. With more advanced disease ulcers become large, often are linear, and typically run longitudinally down the length of the colon. Undermining of nonulcerated mucosa gives rise to the characteristic "cobblestone" appearance of surface nodularity and bumps in Crohn's disease (Color Plate 3). Important features are that the distribution of lesions is asymmetric in its circumferential distribution and often segmental in its longitudinal distribution. Strictures (Color Plate 19) may develop. Despite having features distinct from ulcerative colitis (Table 7.3), 15% of patients with inflammatory bowel disease have a nonspecific colitis that cannot be clearly labelled as Crohn's disease versus ulcerative colitis.

## ISCHEMIC COLITIS

The arterial blood supply to the right colon derives from the superior mesenteric artery (right colic branch; Fig. 7.13). The descending

**Table 7.3** *Clinical and Endoscopic Features of Ulcerative Colitis Versus Crohn's Disease*

|  | *Ulcerative Colitis* | *Crohn's Disease* |
| --- | --- | --- |
| Rectal bleeding | Usually | Sometimes |
| Tenesmus | Usually | Sometimes |
| Diarrhea | Typical | Common |
| Abdominal pain | Yes | Yes |
| Involves rectum | Always | Sometimes |
| Skip lesions | Never | Characteristic |
| Perianal fistulae | Rare | Common |
| Mucosa normal between ulcers | No | Frequently |
| Cobblestoning | No | Typical |
| Filiform pseudopolyps | Yes | Rare |
| Strictures | Uncommon | Typical |

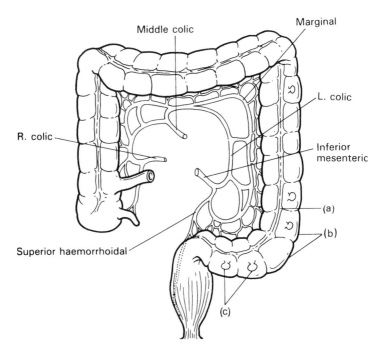

**Fig. 7.13** *Anatomy of the colon, including arterial supply: (A) teniae, (B) sacculations, and (C) appendices epiploica. (Reprinted by permission from Bevan PG, Donovan IA. Handbook of general surgery. Oxford: Blackwell Science, 1992.)*

and sigmoid colons are supplied by the inferior mesenteric artery. The rectum is supplied by the inferior mesenteric artery and by vessels derived from the iliac arteries. Because the syndrome of ischemic colitis generally results from insufficiency of the inferior mesenteric artery, ischemic colitis usually involves the left colon. Classically the splenic flexure is involved, as this area is the "watershed" between the superior and inferior mesenteric artery circulation (i.e., it is at the extreme periphery of both circulations). The rectum is typically spared because of its dual blood supply.

In approximately 80% of cases the affected area in ischemic colitis is within the reach of a 60-cm flexible sigmoidoscope. Thus, flexible sigmoidoscopy can be used to evaluate and follow patients with ischemic colitis. However, when ischemia is suspected and flexible sigmoidoscopy is negative, either colonoscopy or barium enema should be performed to rule out a more proximal distribution of ischemic colitis.

The endoscopic findings of ischemic colitis depend on the stage at which the patient is evaluated. In the initial symptomatic stage the affected areas show patchy edema and hyperemic mucosa alternating with areas that appear to be blanched. The hyperemic areas are friable. Over the following 1 to 3 days superficial ulcerations develop and pinpoint petechiae or occasionally bluish submucosal blebs appear. The petechiae or submucosal blebs are manifestations of submucosal bleeding. In the final stage the ulcers extend to involve more of the mucosal surface, and may develop a longitudinal appearance that is similar to Crohn's disease. Classically these ulcers may occupy only one wall of the colon (Color Plate 20).

Over the course of 6 to 8 weeks most patients will have complete healing. However, some patients heal with formation of strictures (Fig. 7.14), which may or may not be symptomatic.

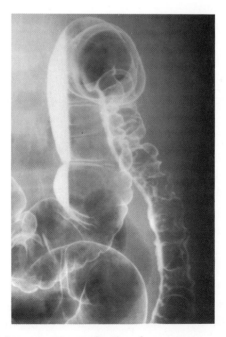

**Fig. 7.14** *A barium enema examination demonstrates a postischemic stricture of the left colon. (Courtesy Dr John Lappas.)*

The diagnosis of ischemic colitis is confirmed by a compatible clinical and endoscopic or radiographic appearance. The combination of new-onset lower abdominal pain, diarrhea, and overt or occult rectal bleeding in an elderly patient with atherosclerotic disease is highly suggestive. If thumb printing (colon wall edema corresponding to submucosal blebs at sigmoidoscopy) is present on plain radiographs, the diagnosis is essentially certain. If necessary, either endoscopy or barium enema can be used to confirm the diagnosis. Angiography, essential to the diagnosis of mesenteric ischemia, has no meaningful role in the diagnosis of ischemic colitis.

Patients are in general managed with gut rest until their discomfort resolves. If there is low-grade fever or elevation of the white blood cell count, then systemic antibiotics directed toward gut flora are appropriate. Serial abdominal examinations are performed; if the patient develops peritoneal findings, full-thickness necrosis of the colon has occurred. Such patients should be referred for segmental colon resection.

### ■ RADIATION COLITIS

Radiation injury to the bowel is essentially an ischemic injury. Patients having endoscopic findings of radiation colitis may be asymptomatic or suffer from constipation, altered bowel habit, abdominal or rectal pain, or rectal bleeding. The characteristic endoscopic finding is numerous spider-like telangiectasias (Color Plate 21). Rectal ulceration and stenoses also may be seen.

Effective therapies for bleeding include Neodymium Yag laser, endoscopic electrocautery, or telangiectasias. Recent reports claim success with rectal administration of formalin and with short chain fatty acid enemas.

### ■ PSEUDOMEMBRANOUS COLITIS

Pseudomembranous colitis should be considered in all patients who develop watery diarrhea within 2 to 3 months of oral or intravenous antibiotics. The syndrome results from overgrowth of a toxin producing *Clostridium difficile*. The diagnosis can now be made with rapid assays of stool for the *C. difficile* antigen or toxin. If the diagnosis must be made quickly, then flexible sigmoidoscopy also is an excellent diagnostic option. The characteristic endoscopic findings are adherent yellow plaques (Color Plate 22) that can become confluent in severe cases. When not confluent, the intervening mucosa appears relatively normal or demonstrates erythema. Patients with mild cases sometimes have endoscopic variants, in which only small plaques surrounded by erythema are seen.

Treatment can be by simple withdrawal of antibiotics or by the administration of cholestyramine in mild cases. Patients with significant symptoms are treated with metronidazole 250 mg four times a day by mouth for 10 days. Severe or refractory cases should be treated with vancomycin 125 mg four times a day by mouth for 10 days. Fifteen percent of patients relapse, and often can be cured by a second course of antibiotics. Patients with multiple relapses are treated successfully with a tapering course of vancomycin (see references).

## MISCELLANEOUS

Patients with portal hypertension will occasionally manifest rectal varices (Color Plate 23). Biopsy can result in severe hemorrhage and must be avoided. Patients taking anthracene cathartics sometimes develop a brownish discoloration to the mucosa called "melanosis coli" (Color Plate 24). Melanosis is a misnomer, because the responsible pigment is lipofuscin. Melanosis can develop within a few months of initiating laxatives and resolve within a few months of discontinuation. Endoscopy texts detail a variety of other lesions that are occasionally or rarely encountered during flexible sigmoidoscopy. Primary care physicians should refer patients to a more experienced endoscopist when lesions of uncertain type are encountered.

## SUMMARY

Good familiarity with the above conditions will allow the examiner to interpret pathology seen at more than 95% of flexible sigmoidoscope examinations. In cases in which unusual findings are encountered, the best course often is referral to a gastroenterologist.

## ▓ RECORDING THE EXAMINATION

The procedure note should include the date, patient identification data, the indication, the model number of the sigmoidoscope, the preparation given, the quality of preparation, the results of external inspection and digital examination, the extent of endoscopic examination, the reason for discontinuation of the examination, the find-

BEST OFFICE IN TOWN

| SIGMOIDOSCOPY REPORT | PATIENT ID |
|---|---|

Date:
Indication:

Screen___ Rectal Bleed___ Abdominal Pain___
Diarrhea___Constipation___Inflammatory Bowel Disease___

Instrument:

Premeds:    None

Preparation: 2 Fleets;  Mg citrate/Fleets;

Prep Quality: Excellent ___ Good ___ Marginal ___ Poor ___

External Inspection:

Digital Examination:

Depth of Exam: _____ cm

Exam Terminated Secondary to:

Complete _____ Discomfort _____ Stool _____

Angulation ____ Polyp Found ____

Mucosal Exam:                 Size   Location
                Polyp        ___   _____
                Polyp        ___   _____
                Polyp        ___   _____
                Diverticulosis: None  Mild  Mod   Severe
                Internal Hemorrhoids: None  Small  Large
                Other: _____
                The examined segments of colon were otherwise normal.
Immediate complications:  None

Biopsies Taken  Yes ____  No ____
Impression:

Plan:                                        _____
                                             BEST DOCTOR IN TOWN

**Fig. 7.15** *Example of a sigmoidoscopy report form.*

ings, whether biopsy specimens were taken, and whether there were immediate complications. Finally, the impression and plan are recorded and the note is signed. An example of a form similar to the one used at Indiana University is shown in Figure 7.15 for your reproduction. Computer programs for generating reports are available from sigmoidoscope manufacturers, but are expensive for office practice.

# Bibliography

▼　▼　▼　▼　▼　▼　▼　▼

Cannon-Albright LA, Skolnick MH, Bishop DT, et al. Common inheritance of susceptibility to colonic adenomatous polyps and associated colorectal cancers. N Engl J Med 1988;318:533–537.

*You have a patient in your office and you're wondering "could this person have a colon polyp"? The presence or absence of colonic symptoms is unlikely to give the answer. Demographic factors such as age are most important. The above study, which was performed using flexible sigmoidoscopy, also showed that male gender and a family history of colorectal cancer were predictive of adenomas. Some, but not all, colonoscopic studies also have shown that family history predicts adenomas.*

Ottenjann R, Burlefinger RJ. Inflammatory bowel diseases. Endoscopy 1992; 24:73–79.

*This article is an excellent review of endoscopic papers on inflammatory bowel disease, including infectious colitis.*

Rex DK, Cummings OW. The controversy regarding distal hyperplastic polyps. Gastrointest Endosc Clin North Am 1993;3:639–648.

*A general consensus now is that a distal hyperplastic polyp is not an indication for colonoscopy, but not all would agree. The above article provides a detailed review of this controversy.*

Scowcroft CW, Sanowski RA, Vzozarek RA. Colonoscopy in ischemic colitis. Gastrointest Endosc 1981;27:156–161.

*This is a classic study on the distribution of endoscopic findings in ischemic colitis. Approximately 80% of patients have disease within reach of a flexible sigmoidoscope. If flexible sigmoidoscopy is negative, one must proceed to colonoscopy or barium enema.*

Tedesco F. Approach to patients with multiple relapses of antibiotic associated pseudomembranous colitis. Am J Gastroenterol 1985;80:867–868.

*If you have a patient with multiple relapses of pseudomembranous colitis, here is the cure! The organism is a spore-forming bacteria, and the spores may not be killed by a single course of antibiotics. Gradual tapering allows the spores to develop and then be killed by the antibiotic. The regimen is vancomycin 125 mg every 6 hours for 1 week, 125 mg every 12 hours for 1 week, 125 mg daily for 1 week, 125 mg every other day for 1 week, and 125 every third day for 2 weeks.*

Tedesco FJ, Corless JK, Brownstein RE. Rectal sparing in antibiotic-associated pseudomembranous colitis: a prospective study. Gastroenterology 1982;83:1250–1260.

*Some authors have advocated colonoscopy as the initial diagnostic endoscopic modality for suspected pseudomembranous colitis. The rationale for such an argument is that some patients have only right-sided pseudomembranes. However, the above prospective evaluation showed that 90% of patients had pseudomembranes within reach of a flexible sigmoidoscope. Therefore, flexible sigmoidoscopy is the preferred initial diagnostic study when an endoscopic procedure is needed.*

Truelove SS, Witts LJ. Cortisone in ulcerative colitis: final report on a therapeutic trial. BMJ 1955;2:1041–1048.

*If you wish to perform flexible sigmoidoscopy in patients with ulcerative colitis, it is essential to know an endoscopic grading system like the one described in the text. However, a clinical grading system is even more important for making therapeutic decisions. The above paper contains the classic clinical grading system for ulcerative colitis. If you know this system it will assist you in tailoring therapy.*

Veidenheimer MC, Roberts PL (eds). Colonic diverticular disease. Oxford: Blackwell Science, 1991.

*If you want to know everything about colonic diverticular disease, look no further.*

# The Endoscopy Asistant

▼  ▼  ▼  ▼  ▼  ▼  ▼  ▼

# 8

## ■ PATIENT CARE

The endoscopy assistant is essential to quality patient care. The assistant is involved in patient care preceding, during, and after the sigmoidoscopy. Initially, the assistant greets the patient in a friendly, relaxed, and professional manner, and escorts the patient to the examination room. The patient is instructed on disrobing and proper gowning (opening in the back) and the assistant attends to the care of the patient's valuables. Preprocedure vital signs are taken and recorded, and the patient is positioned on the examination table. During the examination, the assistant continuously monitors the patient's skin color, respiratory rate, and facial expressions. By standing opposite the endoscopist (Fig. 8.1) the patient's discomfort level is obvious to the assistant, who transmits information regarding discomfort to the endoscopist. The assistant often is the first to observe a problem, such as a vasovagal reaction. Although such episodes are rare during flexible sigmoidoscopy, the assistant is critical for early recognition. The assistant's attention to and reassurance of the patient are very useful in maintaining comfort. After the examination, the assistant can help the patient dress and instructs the patient on postexamination care, including what to expect following the procedure (Table 8.1).

## ■ EQUIPMENT

The assistant is in charge of equipment for the examination. This includes a clean examination table that is locked in position and covered in the center area with absorptive pads (Fig. 8.2). The instru-

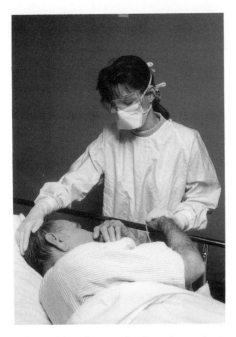

**Fig. 8.1** *Assistant's position for monitoring the patient.*

ment is assembled and attached to the light source, along with the necessary connections for air and water insufflation, as well as for suction. The assistant turns on the instrument prior to the examination and checks that all parts are functioning properly. Necessary supplies are neatly arranged and located so that during the examination, gauze swabs, water-flusher, gloves, camera, lubricant, a pail for soiled swabs, and biopsy forceps are all within reach. Other supplies, such as specimen jars, specimen carriers, labels, and needles to transfer biopsy tissue to the specimen jars, must be close at hand. Although medications are rarely used for flexible sigmoidoscopy, a tray with a tourniquet, alcohol swabs, and butterfly needles should be available.

## ■ DURING THE EXAMINATION

During flexible sigmoidoscopy, the patient lies on an examination table in the left lateral recumbent position. The assistant stands fac-

**Table 8.1** *Instructions Following Flexible Sigmoidoscopy Examination*

---

☐ Inpatient ☐ Outpatient

Diet

1. You may resume your normal diet after the examination unless directed otherwise.
2. Special diet instructions: _____

Special instructions

1. Biopsy specimens were taken, polyps were removed. You should avoid aspirin or arthritis medications (Advil, Motrin, Clinoril, etc) for 14 days to lessen the risk of any postprocedure bleeding. Tylenol or medications containing acetaminophen are okay.
2. You will be notified of biopsy results by phone or mail.
3. Notify us immediately if you notice any of the following:
   a. Rectal bleeding equalling more than 3–4 tablespoons during the next 10 days.
   b. Shaking, chills, or fever over 100°F within 3–5 days.
   c. Severe abdominal pain within the next 3–5 days. (Some discomfort, "gas," and bloating are normal.)
4. Return clinic appointment is scheduled for: _____
   Return procedural appointment is scheduled for: _____
5. Prescriptions given: _____
6. Additional instructions: _____
   _____
7. Call (xxx) xxx-xxxx between 8:00 AM and 5:00 PM for any questions or problems. After 5:00 PM or on weekends or holidays, call (xxx) xxx-xxxx.

These instructions have been reviewed with me: _____
                                              Patient Signature

_____
    Nurse or Physician Signature

---

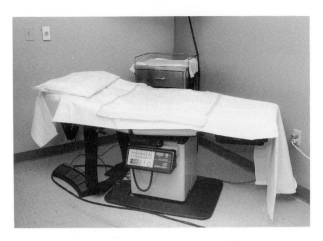

**Fig. 8.2** *The examination table prepared for the patient.*

ing the patient's head, on the opposite side of the table from the endoscopist. From this position, the endoscopic assistant monitors the patient's status. During insertion, the assistant may be asked to hold the instrument near the rectum to prevent the patient from expelling the instrument (see Chapter 6). Lubricant may be applied to the instrument to ease anal passage. A water-flush through the biopsy channel can be given to wash the colon wall and improve visibility. A supply of nonsterile 4″ × 4″ pads or washcloths should be available to keep the instrument shaft and physician's hands clean. Occasionally, during flexible sigmoidoscopy, the assistant applies abdominal pressure to externally splint the instrument to limit sigmoid looping.

The assistant's help is necessary when taking biopsy specimens. Holding the forceps closed with one hand, the assistant hands the forceps tip to the endoscopist for advancement into the biopsy channel. When instructed, the assistant opens and closes the forceps tips. Once biopsy specimens have been retrieved from the colon, the forceps are opened outside the patient and the tissue is extracted using a needle. The tissue is then placed on a carrier by the assistant and then in a bottle containing formalin (see Chapter 6). The bottle is

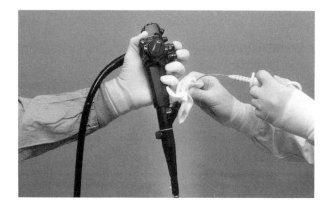

**Fig. 8.3** *Pulling the forceps out while covering the biopsy/suction with gauze.*

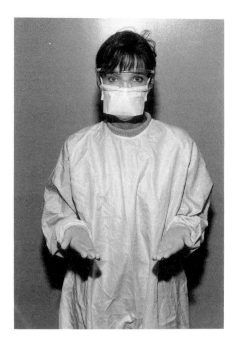

**Fig. 8.4** *Both the assistant and examiner should follow universal precaution (waterproof gown, goggles, mask, and gloves).*

labeled with the patient's name and the location in the colon from which it was taken.

## ■ MISCELLANEOUS DUTIES

The assistant must protect him or herself and the endoscopist from exposure to infection. The assistant, like the endoscopist, wears gloves at all times during the examination and following the procedure during handling of contaminated equipment. When biopsies are performed, holding a nonsterile gauze sponge over the biopsy channel and sliding the forceps through the gauze prevents fluid from being splashed onto the endoscopist or assistant (Fig. 8.3). Both members of the endoscopy team should wear waterproof gowns (Fig. 8.4), which are changed after each procedure.

The assistant should keep a logbook of patients examined, whether biopsies were obtained or photographs taken, and which instruments were used. The assistant must maintain the equipment inventory, including biopsy forceps, cleaning brushes, spare air-water valves, camera film, and lamps for the light source.

The American Society of Gastrointestinal Assistants supports and educates gastrointestinal assistants. This organization is a valuable resource for education of assistants in the technique and standards of endoscopic practice.

# Cleaning and Disinfection

▼    ▼    ▼    ▼    ▼    ▼    ▼    ▼

# 9

O NCE AN examination is completed, there are two distinct steps in preparing the instrument for the next examination. These are cleaning and disinfection. Cleaning implies the mechanical and/or enzymatic removal of debris from the external surface of the sigmoidoscope and the internal channels. Disinfection involves soaking the external surface of the instrument and its internal channels in a cidal solution, and is the subject of the next section of this chapter. It is very important when the sigmoidoscope is purchased to have the manufacturers' representative review the cleaning process with both you and your assistant. Meticulous attention to proper cleaning and disinfection is very important for prolonging the life of the sigmoidoscope, in addition to preventing transmission of infection between patients.

## ■ CLEANING

The tools needed for cleaning are two deep sinks or large basins (Fig. 9.1), the cleaning brushes provided by the sigmoidoscope manufacturer, 70% isopropyl alcohol, cotton-tipped applicators, a toothbrush, and an adequate suction source. Listed below are the recommended steps for cleaning. However, the manufacturer's specific instructions should be followed, and the manufacturer generally supplies many of the essential tools needed for cleaning.

1. Mechanical cleansing is begun immediately after the procedure, before secretions can begin to dry. Suction water through the instrument to remove large debris particles. With the endoscope still attached to the light source, the water bottle is disconnected

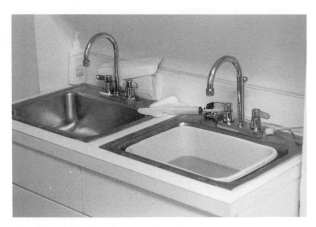

**Fig. 9.1** *Double sinks for cleaning and disinfection.*

from the endoscope and a gloved finger is placed over the air-water inlet until bubbles are blowing out the endoscope tip. This helps clear debris from the air/water channel.

2. Place the insertion tube in a basin or sink filled with cleaning solution. This can be either warm soapy water or a dilution of a commercially available enzymatic cleaning solution. (Ask the manufacturer's representative for names of appropriate enzymatic cleaning solutions). The soapy water or enzymatic cleaning solution is aspirated through the suction-biopsy channel and the shaft of the instrument is wiped down with the cleaning solution using nonsterile 4″ × 4″ gauze pads.

3. Remove the inlet valves to the suction and air-water channels and the biopsy inlet and the hood from the distal tip (from some models) of the instrument shaft (Fig. 9.2). Wash these in the cleaning solution and rinse them in tap water for placement in the disinfectant solution. Use the cotton-tipped applicators to wipe debris from the biopsy channel inlet near the control head and the exit on the distal tip. Use the cleaning brush supplied by the manufacturer to brush the entire length of both the insertion tube and the umbilical cord (Fig. 9.3). After brushing these via the suction button, pass the cleaning brush down through the inlet valve to the suction channel (Fig. 9.4). If the instrument

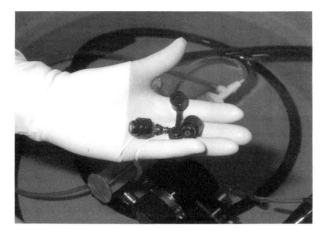

**Fig. 9.2** *Valves and suction inlet cover removed for cleaning and disinfection.*

is not fully immersible, wipe the handle and ocular lens with 70% alcohol solution.

4. Suction an additional 200 mL of soapy water or cleaning solution through the instrument and then immerse the insertion tube into a basin or sink of warm clean tap water. Suction several

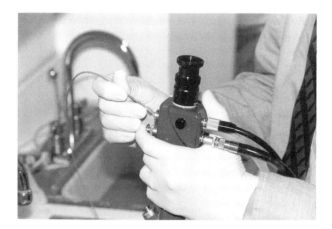

**Fig. 9.3** *Running the cleaning brush down the suction channel.*

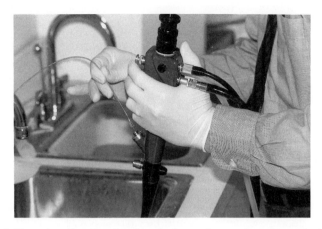

**Fig. 9.4** *Running the cleaning brush down the suction channel via the biopsy inlet.*

hundred milliliters of water through the distal tip and again wipe the instrument off with a clean washcloth.

5. If reusable biopsy forceps were used during the procedure clean them also in the warm soapy water or enzymatic cleaning solution. A washcloth is then used to clean the handle and the coils. The toothbrush may be used to clean the open forceps. Finally, rinse the forceps in clean water and they also are ready for disinfection. Despite these steps, clearing the coils of the forceps of debris can be difficult. Use of an ultrasonic cleaner after mechanical cleaning will help dislodge small particles.

## ■ DISINFECTION

Sterilization of the instrument is not necessary for prevention of transmission of infection. Disinfection is adequate and can be accomplished by manual methods or by the use of automatic disinfecting machines. These machines use either glutaraldehyde, hydrogen peroxide, or peracetic acid as the disinfectant or disinfectant-sterilization agent. The least expensive of these machines is approximately $10,000, making them generally not cost-effective for use in a primary care office practice. In office practice disinfection usually is accomplished by manual methods. Manual methods generally use 2% glutaraldehyde-based solutions as the disinfecting agent. Glutaraldehyde is toxic and can cause a variety of allergic, dermatologic, and pulmonary symptoms. In addition, the material may be carcinogenic. Therefore, it must be handled with respect. Guidelines for the safe use of glutaraldehyde by health care workers are listed below (adapted from Cowan et al. Gut 1993;34:1641–1645):

- Local exhaust ventilation must be used to control glutaraldehyde vapor. Extracted air may be discharged to the atmosphere or passed over special absorbent filters and recirculated. Regular testing and record maintenance is required.
- Endoscope cleaning should be carried out in a designated room equipped with control measures to keep the glutaraldehyde vapor level below 0.2 ppm (preferably below 0.1 ppm).
- Protective equipment should include sterile rubber gloves, apron, chemical-grade eye protection, and respiratory protective equipment.
- Monitoring of atmospheric glutaraldehyde should be by a competent person, preferably by a filtration technique, the commercially available meters being less reliable.
- Health surveillance of staff is mandatory; health records must be maintained for 30 years.

Glutaraldehyde in a 2% solution is a very effective disinfectant. A 20-minute soak is effective in eradicating bacteria, the human immunodeficiency virus, and hepatitis viruses. Longer soaks may be necessary for effective killing of tuberculosis, but a 20-minute soak is currently considered adequate in clinical practice. After completing the soak, it is very important to rinse the glutaraldehyde completely from the endoscope. Failure to do this may result in some glutaraldehyde entering the colon during the next examination, where it can cause a toxic hemorrhagic colitis.

*Steps for Disinfection*

1. Most manufacturers sell inexpensive trays for disinfection of the sigmoidoscope. These trays often are convenient and save on the volume of disinfectant needed. The sigmoidoscope manu-

facturer generally will provide an attachment to be used for filling all the endoscope channels with the disinfecting solution. These cleaning attachments are inserted over the openings to the air-water and suction buttons after removing the valves (Fig. 9.5). The manufacturers' instruction should then be followed to fill all the channels with the disinfecting solution (Fig. 9.6).

2. After filling the channels the instrument shaft is placed in the disinfecting solution. If the instrument is immersible, the entire instrument is placed in the disinfecting solution. The duration of the soak is 20 minutes.

3. When the disinfectant soak is completed either the insertion tube or the entire scope in the case of immersible instruments is placed into a basin containing tap water and 200 to 300 mL of 70% isopropyl alcohol. This solution should be sucked through the distal tip of the scope, used to wipe down the instrument, and to blow out the air water channel. After extensive flushing of the instrument, compressed air can be used to fully blow out the channels. After the last procedure of the day, it is helpful to fill the channels with 70% isopropyl alcohol and then blow them out with compressed air. The use of alcohol

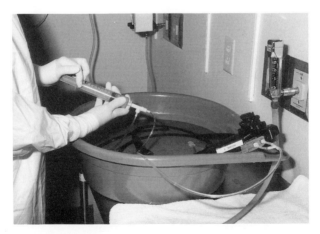

**Fig. 9.5** *The attachment to the air water and suction valves for disinfection of an Olympus sigmoidoscope.*

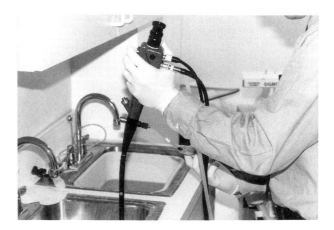

**Fig. 9.6** *Loading disinfectant into the accessory air/water channel.*

facilitates complete drying of the instrument, which will help prevent growth of organisms during overnight storage. As an alternative to compressed air, the instrument can be reattached to the light source and the air water channel can be blown out by holding a gloved finger over the inlet for the water bottle. Finally, the distal tip hood and valve over the suction channel inlet are rinsed, dried, and reattached to the endoscope.

# Bibliography

▼    ▼    ▼    ▼    ▼    ▼    ▼    ▼

Cowan RE, Manning AP, Ayliffe GAJ, et al. Aldehyde disinfectants in health and endoscopy. Gut 1993;34:1641–1645.

*This article makes specific recommendations for the safe use of glutaraldehyde in endoscope disinfection. The article states that manual disinfecting in trays, basins or buckets is inadequate, but this recommendation is not practical for many primary care office practices.*

Duante L, Zulty JC, Israel E, et al. Investigation of an outbreak of bloody diarrhea: association with endoscopic cleaning solution and demonstration of lesions in an animal model. Am J Med 1992;92:476–480.

*In this study a clinic performing screening flexible sigmoidoscopy examinations reported an outbreak of acute symptomatic colitis occurring several hours after the examination. Evaluation revealed that the colitis was the result of failure to clear glutaraldehyde cleaning solution from the sigmoidoscopes. The outbreak started shortly after a new clinical assistant was hired. She apparently felt very rushed and therefore took some short-cuts in preparing the scopes. The paper points out the importance of the examiner maintaining quality control over the cleaning and disinfection process.*

Shields N. A survey of the costs of flexible endoscope cleaning and disinfection. Gastroenterol Nurs 1993;16:53–60.

*Cleaning and disinfection costs approximately $40 per instrument. There is little cost differential between automatic washers and hand-cleaning methods. Staff costs accounted for the largest single component of overall costs. Cleaning-related damage to the instruments contributed significantly to the costs.*

Tremain S, Orientale E, Rodney W. Cleaning, disinfection, and sterilization of gastrointestinal endoscopes: approaches in the office. J Fam Pract 1991: 32:300–305.

*Strict attention to cleaning and disinfection of endoscopes is necessary. Automated washing machines are expensive and no better in efficacy and safety than hand-washing methods.*

# Complictions

▼    ▼    ▼    ▼    ▼    ▼    ▼    ▼

## 10

C OMPLICATIONS resulting from flexible sigmoidoscopy are rare. Since sigmoidoscopy usually is performed without sedation and since therapeutics such as polypectomy and cautery usually are performed at colonoscopy, many of the complications associated with colonoscopy do not apply. Still, an understanding of potential complications is essential so that they can be avoided or rapidly recognized and treated.

Hemodynamic changes are the most common complication occurring during sigmoidoscopy. Tachycardia and hypertension usually relate to anxiety and are not considered complications. Vasovagal reactions occur in approximately 1% of examinations and are characterized by diaphoresis, bradycardia, and hypotension. Syncope has been reported in 0.3% of examinations. The mechanism behind the vasovagal reaction is unknown, but generally is considered to be pain from mesenteric stretching and/or colonic distention by air. Vasovagal reactions may be more common in moderate to severe diverticular disease, presumably because more air distention is often used for sigmoidoscope advancement in these patients.

Colonic perforation is the most serious complication of sigmoidoscopy, occurring at a rate of one in 10,000 examinations. The risk is certainly higher early in the examiner's experience and probably becomes negligible in the hands of an experienced examiner.

Although rare, perforation (along with failure to diagnose cancer) is quite likely to result in a malpractice suit. Failure to recognize and promptly treat a perforation is as serious an error as the perforation itself. Perforation by a primary care physician should always result in immediate consultation with a surgeon.

The most common perforation is the free intraperitoneal perfo-ration. It may be recognized by visualization of a hole in the colonic wall during the examination, and passage of the scope through this hole results in visualization of omentum, bowel serosa, and other peritoneal structures. In some cases, free perforation is recognized only after the procedure is completed. Accompanying findings include pneumoperitoneum on radiographs (Fig. 10.1), abdominal pain, fever, and peritoneal findings on examination. Free perfora-tion, particularly if the peritoneum is visualized during the proce-dure, should be treated surgically.

Rarely patients develop intraperitoneal air after the procedure in the absence of fever and peritoneal signs and with only mild abdominal pain. This condition has been called "benign pneumo-peritoneum." Such patients may be managed conservatively, but surgical consultation is mandatory.

Rectal perforation or retroperitoneal perforation of the descend-ing colon may present without free intraperitoneal air. These patients may develop dramatic retroperitoneal air (Fig. 10.2) on radi-

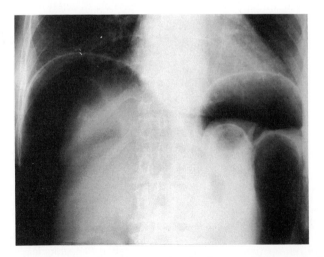

**Fig. 10.1** *Free intraperitoneal air under diaphragms following endo-scopic perforation of the sigmoid during flexible sigmoidoscopy. (Cour-tesy of Dr John Lappas.)*

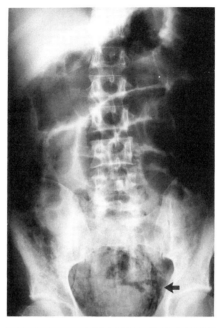

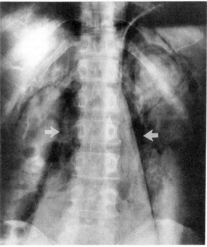

**Fig. 10.2** *Examples of retroperitoneal air dissection (see arrows) following rectal perforation. (A) An ileus pattern is accompanied by a mottled gas pattern (arrow) from retroperitoneal gas in the pelvis following perforation of the rectum by a rigid sigmoidoscope (arrow). (B) Retroperitoneal gas outlines the psoas muscles (arrows) and kidneys after perforation by an enema tip. (Courtesy of Dr John Lappas.)*

ographs, with extension into the mediastinum or subcutaneous space. If pain and fever are present, surgery should be considered. However, antibiotics, nothing by mouth, and observation often are successful in these patients. Rectal perforation during flexible sigmoidoscopy should be rare. The examples shown in Figure 10.2 occurred from rigid sigmoidoscopy and an enema tip. However, instrumentation (biopsy) forceps and the retroflex maneuver provide opportunity for rectal perforation during flexible sigmoidoscopy, particularly in a diseased rectum.

Perforation occurs most commonly in the sigmoid colon (80% of cases). Errors in advancement involve pushing on diverticular orifices (Fig. 10.3), pushing through bowel damaged or narrowed by ischemia, radiation, or cancer (Fig. 10.4), and pushing against fixed resistance (Fig. 10.5). Fixed resistance results from serosal adhesions or tumor. The mucosal surface in such cases may appear normal. The final mechanism of perforation involves overdistention of the cecum by air insufflation. This is particularly likely if the scope passes a narrowing in the sigmoid (Fig. 10.6). Insufflated air

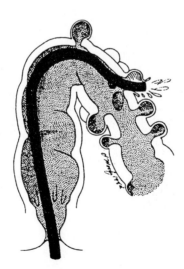

**Fig. 10.3** *Perforation by forceful advancement into a large diverticulum. (Reprinted by permission from Katon RM, Keefe EB, Melnyk CS. Flexible sigmoidoscopy. Orlando: Grune and Stratton, 1985, p. 106.)*

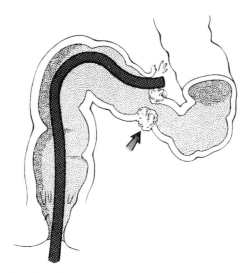

**Fig. 10.4** *Perforation by overly aggressive pressure on a malignant stricture. In this case the scope may suddenly slip to the side and pop through normal wall adjacent to the tumor. (Reprinted by permission from Katon RM, Keefe EB, Melnyk CS. Flexible sigmoidoscopy. Orlando: Grune and Stratton, 1985.)*

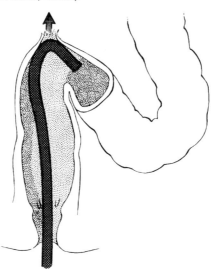

**Fig. 10.5** *Perforation by pushing in areas of fixed resistance. Note that perforation may occur while the lumen is in clear view. (Reprinted by permission from Katon RM, Keefe EB, Melnyk CS. Flexible sigmoidoscopy. Orlando: Grune and Stratton, 1985, p. 107.)*

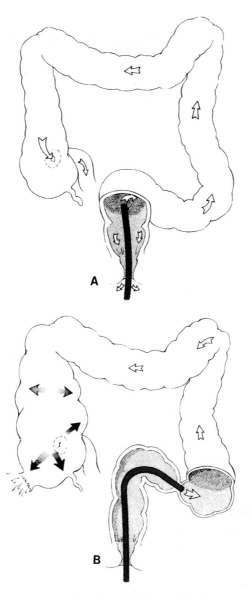

**Fig. 10.6** *Pneumatic perforation. (A) Generally air can escape through the anus and ileocecal valve. (B) The ileocecal valve is competent to air and the sigmoidoscope is impacted in a stricture, preventing insufflated air from escaping to the rectum. (Reprinted by permission from Katon RM, Keefe EB, Melnyk CS. Flexible sigmoidoscopy. Orlando: Grune and Stratton, 1985, p. 109.)*

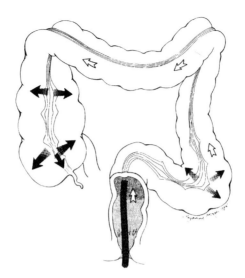

**Fig. 10.7** *Serosal laceration. These tears are most likely to occur along the antimesenteric borders. (Reprinted by permission from Katon RM, Keefe EB, Melnyk CS. Flexible sigmoidoscopy. Orlando: Grune and Stratton, 1985, p. 112.)*

may not be able to escape through the narrowing to the rectum. If the ileocecal valve is competent, the colon may quickly distend with air and the cecum (the thinnest part of the colon) may burst. Localized mesenteric stretching or compartmentalization of air may result in serosal tears without perforation (Fig. 10.7). These patients may be asymptomatic or may develop abdominal pain and distention. Spontaneous resolution of symptoms is the rule.

Transmitted infections are the third most common complication of sigmoidoscopy. Prevention requires meticulous attention to cleaning and disinfection, as discussed in Chapter 9. Recommendations for preventions of endocarditis are given in Chapter 4.

Bleeding during diagnostic flexible sigmoidoscopy is rare. Use of aspirin or nonsteroidal anti-inflammatory drugs is not a contraindication to mucosal biopsies. Therapeutic anticoagulation is a contraindication. In general, the prothrombin time should be 15 seconds or less and the platelet count 50,000 $mm^3$ for mucosal biopsy specimens to be safely taken.

# Bibliography

▼     ▼     ▼     ▼     ▼     ▼     ▼     ▼

Monahan D, Peluso F, Goldner F. Combustible colonic gas levels during flexible sigmoidoscopy and colonoscopy. Gastrointest Endosc 1992;38: 40–43.

*Ten percent of patients undergoing sigmoidoscopy, using a phosphosoda enema as preparation, will have combustible levels of hydrogen and methane gas present. Due to the risk of explosion, electrocautery should not be performed during sigmoidoscopy.*

Spach D, Silverstein F, Stamm W. Transmission of infection by gastrointestinal endoscopy and bronchoscopy. Ann Intern Med 1993;118:117–128.

*The most common infections transmitted by improperly cleaned instruments include* Salmonella *sp,* Pseudomonas *sp, and* Mycobacterium *sp. Two hundred eighty-one cases of endoscope-associated transmission are reviewed.*

Traul D, Davis G, Pollack J, et al. Flexible fiberoptic sigmoidoscopy—the Monroe Clinic experience. A prospective study of 5000 examinations. Dis Colon Rectum 1983;26:161–166.

*Syncope was the most common complication.*

# Index

▼   ▼   ▼   ▼   ▼   ▼   ▼   ▼